"**The Building** Energy book employs the ⟨...⟩ ⟨...⟩ ⟨...⟩ ⟨...⟩ ⟨...⟩ impact valuable health information and tech⟨...⟩ ⟨...⟩ upon its readers. It is the use of this very simply approach to discussing what can be a complicated topic, nutrition, that makes me recommend this book to my clients. **Building Energy** delivers what it promises, without confusing the reader, it empowers the reader! Two thumbs up!"

PHYLLIS REID-JARVIS
Registered Dietician and owner of
PRJ Consulting

"**Building Energy** is a complete and comprehensive 'how to guide' to living an energized, vital life. It is overflowing with the knowledge and tools needed to making successful, long lasting lifestyle changes. I found the book to be 'action oriented' and empowering."

ROBIN ANDERSON
Registered Dietician and owner of
Steps to Wellness Nutrition Consulting

"**Building Energy** has helped my energy levels immensely! I am in an administrative position and sit most of my day, so, the stretch at your desk exercises were very helpful. I have also incorporated brief exercise breaks into my day rather than the traditional coffee breaks, I now have energy to spare. I am also working on increasing my water intake and decreasing the caffeine fix I used to need. Thanks so much for my new found energy!

MARIE HIEBERT
Executive Director
Alberta Fencing Association

Building Energy

A complete guide to finding a new energized you!

Bev Richardson and Wendy Bodnar

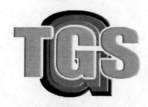

The Growth Shop

"Teaching Growth Solutions"

www.thegrowthshop.com

ISBN 0-7414-1660-3

Published by:

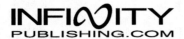

519 West Lancaster Avenue
Haverford, PA 19041-1413
Info@buybooksontheweb.com
www.buybooksontheweb.com
Toll-free (877) BUY BOOK
Local Phone (610) 520-2500
Fax (610) 519-0261

Printed in the United States of America

Printed on Recycled Paper

Published October 2003

TABLE OF CONTENTS

Foreword

Building Energy is based on the belief that most people today face a personal "energy crisis", and are too fatigued to enjoy life to the fullest. The increased levels of stress and chronic illness that are by-products of our society confirm this. Time and work pressures, greater reliance on technology, increased availability of convenience and fast foods, and decreased opportunities for physical activity have led to alarming increases in obesity and Type 2 diabetes. It is difficult, however, to reach the majority of North Americans whose lifestyles are not sufficiently healthy. **Building Energy** is one resource that can aid in this goal, by motivating and assisting everyone to make healthy lifestyle choices.

We are overloaded with information about health: in magazines, on the World Wide Web and on television. It is often difficult to sift through this information, and find those items that are directly helpful in our lives. **Building Energy** translates theory and research into information that is personally relevant to healthy lifestyle choices. A major strength of the workbook is its *hands-on approach*. Not just another compilation of information, it provides many useful worksheets and resources that will help you make lifestyle changes. The mother/daughter authors, Bev Richardson and Wendy Bodnar, have put together just the right mix of facts and practical tips for applying this information in your life. The book is based on many years of stress management and building energy courses offered by the authors. Wendy's company, **The Growth Shop**, is dedicated to personal and professional growth. She has a background in physical education, and is well respected in the fitness community. Bev has considerable experience in adult education. The authors have consulted Registered Dietitians to complement their expertise.

Building Energy is designed to help you increase your energy levels. Unlike many programs that emphasize losing weight or improving fitness levels, this book focuses on *helping you feel better*. **Building Energy** is organized in five sections: **E**nergy/Everyone, **N**utrition, **E**xercise, **R**est, and **G**oals for **Y**ou – **ENERGY!** Each section gives readers the knowledge necessary to make energy boosting choices in their daily lives. I particularly like the use of worksheets and creating personal lists (e.g. personal energy gains and drains), nutrition quizzes, a physical activity recall, self-assessment of sleep patterns, and a Daily Building Energy Record. All of these tools surpass just knowledge but support implementation on an on-going basis.

The publication of this book is timely, given the increasing negative affects of inactivity, stress, and poor eating habits on our health. Many people are now aware that changing their lifestyle would make them healthier, and give them greater energy to meet each day. Unfortunately, most people don't know *how* to become more active, eat better, or relax. **Building Energy** is an excellent resource to help you begin, and maintain, healthy lifestyle changes.

Elizabeth Ready, Ph.D.
Associate Dean,
Faculty of Physical Education and Recreation Studies,
University of Manitoba

Acknowledgements

It takes many dedicated people to compile a workbook like **Building Energy**. Both Bev and Wendy worked countless hours and followed the principles that they discovered to maintain their energy levels during the many drafts.

We want to thank our resident Registered Dietitian and head cheerleader, Phyllis Reid-Jarvis of PRJ Consulting, for her valuable advice and recommendations on the nutrition section of this workbook. Nancy Hill, a certified Fitness Trainer and Physical Education graduate, not only added her expertise, but her grammatical talents as well. Our initial pilot workshop participants, Phyllis Reid-Jarvis, Nancy Hill, Barb Sawyer, Andrew Jarmus, and Paul Bodnar for their feedback and encouragement. Paul Bodnar spent endless hours editing the written works of this workbook. Monica Richardson, Wendy's daughter, for her gift of drawing and capturing the essence of energy.

Thank you to Dr. Elizabeth Ready for reading the book and agreeing to write a foreword. Her input to the book is invaluable and her words of encouragement are greatly appreciated. Also to those who agreed to read the draft of the book and to give us input and write testimonials, Phyllis, Robin and Marie.

We would also like to thank Jackie Desrocher and Karen Meelker at the Organization and Staff Development Agency of the Civil Service Commission, Government of Manitoba for their support. They had the foresight to see the importance of **Building Energy** for their marketplace and hosted the first full one-day workshop.

Bev and Wendy would like to acknowledge the special men in both of their lives. Bev's husband Jim put up with the hours of research, a messy dining room table, and even trying soya nuts. Wendy's husband Paul read and re-read this workbook ad nauseam. He never tired of the changes, special requests, and regular need for support and back massages.

We would like to thank our publishing company, Infinity Publishing for the wonderful job they have done putting the book you hold together.

This book has been a joy to write. Mother and daughter working side by side sharing the research, the excitement, and now an even more special bond.

Introduction

During our many years of researching and teaching stress management courses we discovered that many of our participants were suffering from fatigue. With the ever-changing workplace environment some people found themselves in positions that two or three people once filled. The productivity demand was high and the energy levels became low. This not only affected their work performance, but influenced their personal lives as well. These realizations were confirmed even further by the research of both Canadians and Americans and their health. The obesity levels, Type 2 diabetes, lack of proper sleep, dehydration and general fatigue were reaching alarming numbers. All of this led to **Building Energy**.

We made the decision to begin a quest into the realm of energy and how we could regain the vitality in our lives on a daily basis. How could we eat for energy? How could we help people get a good night's sleep to keep their energy levels high during their busy days? What were our energy drains and how could we minimize them? These were just some the questions that we wanted answers for.

Building Energy is designed to help everyone understand their own energy requirements and is a hands-on workbook to maximize results. In our research, we have found that people accept changes in their lives more easily and with better results when they can write things down and set realistic goals. The energy acronym, *E-Energy is for Everyone, N-Nutrition, E-Exercise, R-Rejuvenation through Rest, G- Goals and Y-You*, was developed by Bev as an instant reminder of the energy builders that this workbook is based upon.

Building Energy is laid out in an easy to read fashion featuring our basic understanding of energy production in the body, how our body can maintain energy and how to avoid things that drain our energy. Each section of the workbook has Wendy's 5 W's: W-Watch what you eat; W- Water, drink a lot of it; W-Walk as often as you can; W-Weights build strength and muscular endurance; and W-Wonderful is how you will feel. These simple exercises will assist the reader in reviewing and making action plans to increase energy. We have organized the *Nutrition* section with the food fuel of choice in preferential order. Carbohydrates are the body's first choice for energy. They, followed by fats and lastly proteins, are easily converted to glucose to be further broken down for energy. The important role of water, vitamins and minerals are also discussed. Energy begets energy! This statement rings true and the *Exercise* section will explain how this works and gives you actual exercises to incorporate into daily living. Our body needs to get proper rest to be at peak energy performance. The *Rejuvenation through Rest* section takes a comprehensive look at how to develop sleep hygiene and some basic do's and don'ts. Finally **Building Energy** addresses our individual commitment and positive attitude toward our energy and vitality in the *Goals and You* section.

It is our hope that you will enjoy the process of reading and writing in your own **Building Energy** workbook. When you follow the basic tips for eating for energy, drinking for energy, exercising for energy and sleeping for energy you will be surprised at your seemingly boundless energy. This will allow you to perform your daily tasks with ease and create an energy reserve to spend with your family and friends. Enjoy your new found energy!

Bev and Wendy

BUILDING

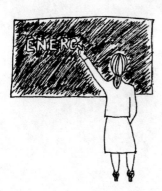

ENERGY
Nutrition
Exercise
Rest and Relaxation
Goals
You

SECTION ONE

ENERGY IS FOR EVERYONE

Keeping healthy, energetic, enjoying your life everyday is up to you!
The ideas and suggestions shared in this book are for everyone.

Note:
This workbook has been put together drawing from a
variety of reputable resources.
It is meant to be a resource and a motivational tool to help you get
started on a more energetic and healthier lifestyle.
It has been read as to accuracy of content by a Registered Dietitian and
a Physical Education Graduate.

*****

It is not meant to take the place of any medical advice.
Should you find you require medical attention,
please see your doctor.

LEARNING OBJECTIVE

After you have read this Section and completed all the exercises, you will

- understand how your body uses and stores fuel and how to ensure you have "the right stuff" to meet your energy needs

BUILDING ENERGY QUIZ

Take time right now to check out how you are doing. Put a corresponding number against each of the following questions. Give yourself

ALWAYS	= 4 points
OFTEN	= 3 points
SOMETIMES	= 2 points
SELDOM	= 1 point
NEVER	= 0 points

If you don't understand a question – leave it blank.

1. I choose complex carbohydrates that are high in fibre. _4_
2. I limit the amount of salt and sugar I eat. _4_
3. I drink no more than 1 alcoholic drink a day. _4_
4. I take a multivitamin each day. _4_
5. I have a job or do other work that I enjoy. _3_
6. I participate in leisure activities and hobbies that I love. _4_
7. I drink 6 to 8 glasses of water every day. _3_
8. I limit the amount of saturated fat I eat each day. _4_
9. I have close friends, relatives, or others whom I can talk to about personal matters and can call on for help when needed. _4_
10. I maintain my weight within 10 pounds of my "ideal weight". _3_
11. I do some form of physical activity for 45 to 60 minutes each day. _0_
12. I do a muscle-toning workout at least 3 times each week. _0_
13. I eat a small portion of protein with every meal and snack. _1_
14. I drink no more than 3 cups of coffee each day. _4_
15. I balance my carbohydrates and protein at every meal and snack. _3_
16. I get a full 8 hours of sleep each night. _4_

TOTAL POINTS _49_

How are you doing at Building Your Energy?

Score of 40+

Way to go! You're putting your knowledge and a healthy lifestyle into building more energy into your life.

Score of 30 – 39

You're working hard on building energy, but there's still room for improvement. Look at areas where you can make some change for the better.

Score of 29 and lower

You may be experiencing a feeling of low energy and some health risks are showing. Look closely at how you are living, and make a serious effort to improve your health and your energy level. Talk to your doctor.

HOW OUR BODY WORKS
AND HOW OUR BODY IS FUELED

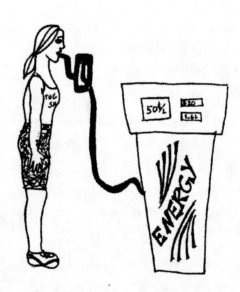

The first "E" in ENERGY stands for <u>E</u>veryone

Your life… Your body…. Your Choices…. Are you loving Life?

Fatigue…… is there an energy crisis? According to the statistics, yes! Why are we so tired? In this book, we will attempt to answer this question and discuss solutions to the energy crisis. We will determine how we can assist our body in the attainment and preservation of energy. Let's start with some basic information. Then we will end this section with a look at the "Energy Equation".

HOW IS THE BODY FUELED?

Before we get into details of discussing the energy equation, we must first look at how the body receives energy and how it uses fuel to create energy. Knowing the basics of how the body works will enable us to discover the best way to fuel the body and to understand how the body will burn this energy to create movement. We must also keep in mind that every "body" is different and unique in its requirements for energy. What works for one person may be a complete disaster for another. So, keep this in mind as we discover the basics of how our body works.

THE FIRST FUEL

Did you know that there is fuel right now available in your cells? As you are sitting in your chair, your body has fuel available for you if you decided to jump up and leap into the air. How is this possible you ask? Well, let's take a look.

In your muscle tissue there is a short-term energy source available without the need for oxygen. This energy source is called ATP (Adenosine Tri-phosphate) and CP (Creatine Phosphate). We give you these large words so you can impress your friends during your next scrabble game. This energy source is just enough to allow you to leap into the air and it lasts for about 10 seconds. Then if you decide to jump up and down many times your amazing body has yet another source of stored energy in the muscle cells. This uses another energy pathway called the lactic acid system. It sounds kind of painful and in fact you'll notice that your muscles will start to send a burning sensation to your brain. That is lactic acid build up in your muscle tissue. What happens is that your muscles have to convert carbohydrates into ATP to provide movement. Without the presence of oxygen, carbohydrates are only partially broken down and that produces lactic acid.

This is why we need to slow down and use our aerobic pathway to get more energy to do lots of smaller jumps. The aerobic pathway is our long-term energy production pathway and it allows us to keep jumping. The fuels in this pathway are both fat and stored carbohydrates. Proteins can be used, but are not the preferred fuel.

FOOD AS FUEL

Our body needs energy from food to keep up the supply of ATP for energy production. We need to continually feed our "machine" good quality food for fuel to make it work. Just like a car engine - it will run smoothly with proper care but with neglect it will need extra tune-ups and maintenance.

The two sources of food in the body that are converted to energy are Carbohydrates and Fats. Proteins are needed to continuously repair and build muscle and tissue.

Food is an indirect fuel source, as it cannot be used directly by our muscles for energy. Instead the energy is released from the breakdown of foodstuffs and used to manufacture a biochemical compound, the ATP we discussed earlier. So, it is very important that we fuel our body correctly with what it needs to perform at peak efficiency.

When our body receives the food that we give it, it has to decide what to do with it. What is used for energy production, what is absorbed as nutrients, what is expelled as waste products and if there is extra - it will be stored as fat. We will discuss this more fully in our nutrition section.

WATER AS FUEL

Water is another absolute source of energy. Water is basic to our very being. Simply put, we can't live without it. Our brain and our body are made up of mostly water. We need water to help our body break down our food enabling us to use the vitamins and minerals needed to build our body's cells.

If we are dehydrated, we become fatigued and lose our energy very quickly. Did you know that the number one cause of fatigue is the lack of water in our body?

PHYSICAL ACTIVITY AS FUEL

We also need physical activity in our lives to keep our energy levels high. If you don't use it, you lose it! Our bodies are designed to move and move them we must. We need to exercise and massage our internal organs, oxygenate our blood and tone our muscles to allow us to live our lives.

To feel energetic, we need to have toned, strong muscles, and the ability to move quickly and with confidence.

REST AS FUEL

Another definite need for energy is sufficient rest; rest for our body and rest for our mind. In this workbook, we will examine sleep and our body's need for rejuvenation – time to rebuild and repair to keep us energized.

Your Notes:

ENERGY

List 5 ways you get your energy up:

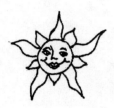

List 5 things that drag you down, depleting your energy:

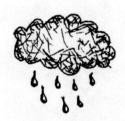

ENERGY GAINS

BREATHE
Our brain and our body must have oxygen to function.

NUTRITION
We need to fuel our bodies with the "right stuff".

WATER
Helps carry needed nutrients and oxygen throughout our body.

PHYSICAL ACTIVITY
Equals energy and we get more energy, through strong muscles and bones.

REST
Rejuvenate your body and your mind.

RELAX
Keep a balanced lifestyle - stay resilient.

JOY
Play, laugh, have fun. Find the 'Bless in the Mess.'

ATTITUDE
Stay positive, it's the key! Plan, set Goals.

The happiest people don't necessarily have the best of everything.
They just make the most of everything that comes their way.

Live life well. It's up to YOU!

ENERGY DRAINS

NEGATIVITY
Drags us *down*
- depression.

POOR FOOD CHOICES
Our bodies can't maintain energy
on junk food.

OVERLOAD
Too many things at one time.
Feeling out of control – stressed.
Leads to confusion, frustration
and exhaustion.

OVERWEIGHT
Weighs us down.
Puts a strain on our backs,
our joints – we're tired!

DEHYDRATION
Body struggles to get nutrients
and oxygen throughout our
body. Retains water as it
thinks we're in a drought.

SEDENTARY
If you don't use it, you lose
it! Muscles get weak, bones
become brittle.

INSOMNIA
Body and mind
cannot rejuvenate
and become
exhausted.

Over use of:
Caffeine
Nicotine
Sugar
Salt
Alcohol

Let's shift these OUT of our lives.

THE ENERGY EQUATION

Your Energy Equation is up to you.

The Energy Gains page shows ways that help us increase our energy.

The Energy Drains page shows how we can be draining our own energy.

So look at how you can build your own ENERGY EQUATION and build more energy into your life.

THE <u>ENERGY EQUATION</u> YOU ARE LOOKING FOR IS:

High Quality Foods + Sufficient Water + Physical Activity + _____ + _____ + _____

MINUS

Low Quality Foods – Dehydration – Lack of Physical Activity – Lack of Sleep, Rest and Relaxation –

_____ – _____ – _____

EQUALS =

"SURPLUS ENERGY"

The Energy Equation

In the next Sections, we will be discovering many ways that our body uses energy and how we can build energy. We also will find out about food and activity that will decrease our energy reserves.

The next few pages give you further information on some of the
ENERGY DRAINS we want to put OUT of our lives.

MORE ENERGY DRAINS

SUGAR - alias sucrose, corn syrup, brown sugar, dextrose and maltose.

Sugar is an empty food, has no nutritional value, is high in calories and can easily cause obesity. We think we can get an energy burst by using sugar as a quick pick-up, like eating a candy bar or having a soft drink. *This will backfire!* Our body uses sugar very rapidly. Sugar will give us a quick pick-up and then a quick letdown. We are often left with a headache, feeling fatigued or irritable and end up feeling hungrier as well.

Refined sugar is absorbed quickly and easily into the bloodstream, elevating the blood sugar level. Our body reacts to this elevated blood sugar level as though it were under attack and releases hormones to assist us in the fight or flight response that we experience during times of stress. It also turns on the mechanisms to store body fat for future fight or flight situations. Both are things we do not want. Reducing our sugar consumption will increase the efficiency of all our digestive organs, resulting in better physical energy in the long run.

SMOKING

We all know that smoking causes cancer, but did you know that smoking is also linked to heart disease and emphysema? In fact smoking is the main cause of preventable death in Canada. When we use tobacco, the effects on our body are immediate. Our pulse increases, our breathing becomes faster and shallower and our circulation begins to drop. A cocktail of over 3,700 substances, many of them that cause cancer, hit our lungs. Poisonous compounds like carbon monoxide, hydrogen cyanide and ammonia gas enter our bloodstream. This all adds up to increased chances of asthma, colds, flu and pneumonia, not to mention the drain on our daily energy needs. We know that some of the chemicals from tobacco smoke actually bind to the oxygen in our bloodstream and decrease the total oxygen available to us.

We need to be able to supply ample oxygen to our brain, muscles and of course our lungs to be healthy and energetic. Please strongly consider stopping smoking to increase your energy. For more information go to www.tobaccofact.org.

CAFFEINE - has addictive properties.

Caffeine stimulates the nervous system, the heart and the respiratory system, and also acts as a diuretic. As a diuretic, caffeine washes water-soluble vitamins (C+B -Complex) out of the body. This compounds the effects of stress by depleting needed nutrients. Caffeine also pulls needed calcium from our bones.

The severity of the symptoms depends on how much is consumed. One cup of strong coffee can extend its influence on the body for up to seven hours, with its peak stimulant effect occurring between two to four hours. It is suggested not to have caffeine after supper because its stimulant effect can disturb our sleep. Two and one half cups of coffee can cause abnormal heart rhythm and increase our heart rate due to the adrenaline in the system. This is why we feel such a rush from caffeine products. The liver must overcompensate to keep the caffeine from affecting our heart, and overall, this depletes our energy. Caffeine can also stimulate our appetite. According to Rick Gallop in his book "The Glycemic Index Diet" caffeine: ".... does lead to increased insulin production, which reduces your blood sugar levels and makes you feel hungry." Excess caffeine is known to aggravate stomach ulcers, insomnia, chest pain, nausea, flushing, racing pulse, headache, irritability and restlessness.

There is still a lot of discussion on the benefits or harm coffee may have on our body. The one thing we know for sure is that coffee has no nutrient value. To be on the safe side, limit yourself to 2-4 cups and drink them earlier in the day.

Sources of Caffeine – Health Canada Recommends no more that 400-450 mg daily

Item	Amount	Mg. Caffeine
Coffee	6 oz cup – filter drip	110-180 mg
	6 oz cup – instant	60-90 mg
Tea	6 oz cup – weak	20-45 mg
	6 oz cup – strong	79-110 mg
Colas	1 10 oz can	22-50 mg
Chocolate	8 oz glass milk	2-7 mg
	2 oz dark chocolate	40-50 mg
	2 oz light chocolate	3-20 mg

ALCOHOL

Just three ounces of alcohol slows down our body's ability to burn fat by about one third. An alcoholic drink has 7 calories per gram – close to fat's 9 calories per gram. Just one ounce of pure alcohol is the equivalent of about one-half an ounce of dietary fat. So, if we drink 2 drinks of beer, cocktails or wine, we are consuming the equivalent of one full ounce of dietary fat. Alcohol also increases our appetite, easily adding up to 350 calories at a meal. "Alcohol is easily metabolized by the body which means increased insulin production, a drop in blood sugar levels and demand from the body for more alcohol or food to boost those sagging sugar levels" (from The Glycemic Index Diet, Rick Gallop). Health gains from having a drink or two each day may be negated by our increased appetites and calorie intake.

Fat gained from alcohol goes directly to the abdomen. Research shows that those who had two drinks per day had the largest waist to hip ratio measurements, which is a direct measurement of health.

SALT - our body needs salt but try not to have more than 2,400 mg of sodium (1 ¼ teaspoons of salt) per day.

We likely get sufficient salt from the foods we eat. In fact it's easier to get too much than too little. Salt is a stimulant. It raises our blood pressure and causes an imbalance in our body. In order to equalize this imbalance our body has to sweat to remove the excess salt. This leads to a quick drop in sodium and causes a depressed, low energy feeling.

Let's watch the amount of highly salted foods we choose, i.e. processed food, snacks, some canned soups, pickles, etc. Watch how much we add while cooking and while eating. If high blood pressure runs in our family – it is especially important for us to watch our sodium intake. "Learn to check labels. Try to eat foods with less than 200 mg of sodium per serving, and definitely avoid those extremely high-sodium foods with more than 800 mg per serving", says researcher Lawrence J. Appel, MD, MPH, of John Hopkins Medical Institutions.

FOOD ADDITIVES, HIGHLY PROCESSED FOODS - avoid as much as possible.

The prevalence of known and suspected carcinogenic elements in artificial colours, additives, preservatives and other processed chemicals is well established. Nitrates, linked as a factor in cancer of the colon, are found in bacon, sausage and luncheon meats.

Highly processed foods have less nutritional *value* because many desirable components have been processed out of them. These same foods are then "enriched" or "preserved" with additives. Over time, the extra work our body must do in dealing with these additives takes a toll on our liver, which must break down, detoxify, or store the unusable substances found in processed foods.

MY NOTES:

MY NOTES:

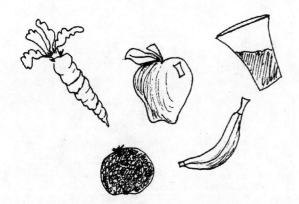

BUILDING

Energy
NUTRITION
Exercise
Rest and Relaxation
Goals
You

SECTION TWO

NUTRITION

FOOD AND WATER AS FUEL

Two main sources of energy are FOOD and WATER.

LEARNING OBJECTIVES

After you have read this Section and completed all the exercises, you will

- understand how your body uses and stores fuel and how to ensure you have "the right stuff" to meet your energy needs
- recognize the nutritional value of food and how your food fuels your energy levels
- recognize dehydration and know why and how much water your body needs to maintain your energy levels
- have information to enable you to make quality choices to maintain general good health and energy by ensuring you get the vitamins and minerals you need

FOOD – FUEL FOR ENERGY

You are what you EAT.

Making good food choices is fundamental to our good health and our energy levels. Eating a nutritious, well balanced diet is crucial to our body's growth and maintenance, protection from many different diseases and to our energy levels. Our food choices can help protect us from heart disease, stroke, osteoporosis, many forms of cancer, high blood pressure, and diabetes just to name a few.

We want to get the majority of our nutrients from the food we eat. We know, however, that with our busy lives, and perhaps some poor eating habits, we are not always getting all the nutrients that we need every day. As we age, our stomach acid production falls which makes nutrient absorption more difficult. So, even though we know that supplements cannot and are not meant to replace our food, we come to the conclusion that there is a real place in our lives to add a good vitamin and mineral supplement to our diet.

We also know that any kind of fad diets, and we've likely all tried at least one, result in only a short-term weight loss. The result of dieting creates a loss of muscle tissue and a gain of fat tissue. We may weigh less because fat tissue weighs less than muscle tissue. Any time we deprive our bodies of food, the very fuel it needs, it thinks we are facing starvation and quickly puts the fat storing machine into high gear. This is an evolutionary mechanism of the feast or famine cycle. All the research agrees that any kind of "dieting" is out. Dieting makes us more susceptible to disease and, in the long run, makes us fatter.

How can we best maintain ourselves? By consistently making good food choices! Our main fuels from food sources are complex carbohydrates, selected fats and quality proteins. Each of these types of foods provides calories – or food energy for our bodies to function every day. In each day of our lives, our body requires a certain amount of calories to survive and thrive. The amount needed is dependent on our sex, height, weight and energy expenditure. Carbohydrates provide 4 calories per gram, fats provide 9 calories and proteins provide 4 calories per gram. You can see that fats more than double the other two.

REVISITING THE BASICS

For our continued good health, it is important to be aware of our nutritional needs. We will be concentrating on how to make effective food choices to build and maintain our energy levels and meet our body's nutritional requirements. We will look at what to choose, how much to choose and how often to eat to sustain our energy all day long.

We want to remind you of some of the basics of nutrition found in the Food Guide (see the next page). In the Food Guide please note the portion sizes that count for one serving, also note the number of servings recommended. The number of servings varies according to our age, whether we are male or female, our body size and our activity level. You choose the number of servings that is right for you.

THE FOOD GUIDE

Remember serving sizes are important. They vary, and we choose what is right for our age, our gender, our body size, and our activity level.

GRAIN PRODUCTS 5-12 servings each day
Mostly carbohydrates – this is your largest food source/your base.

1 serving size	2 servings
1 slice of whole wheat bread	1 bran muffin
30 g /1 oz cold cereal	1 pita
175 ml/ ¾ cup hot cereal	1 bagel
	1 bun
	240 ml/1cup rice or pasta

VEGETABLES AND FRUITS   5 to 10 SERVINGS EACH DAY
Mostly carbohydrates

1 serving size
1 small box of raisins
1 medium size of any vegetable or fruit
125 ml/ ½ cup fresh/frozen/canned fruit or vegetable
250 ml/1 cup salad
125 ml/ ½ cup of juice

MILK PRODUCTS   2-4 SERVINGS EACH DAY
Mostly Protein

½ serving size	1 serving size
125 ml/ ½ cup frozen fruit/ icemilk/yogurt	50 g/ 3"x 1"x 1" cube of cheese
125 ml/ ½ cup pudding	175 g/ ¾ cup of yogurt
250 ml/ 1 cup cottage cheese	50 g/ 2 slices processed cheese
175 ml/ ¾ cup ice cream	250 ml/ 1 cup milk (1%, 2%, or skim)

MEAT AND ALTERNATIVES 2 –3 SERVINGS EACH DAY
Mostly Protein

1 serving size
50 – 100 g/ 2oz – 5 oz meat, poultry or fish
30 ml/ 2 tbsp. peanut butter
125 – 250 ml/ ½ - 1 cup beans
50 – 100 g/ 1/3 – 2/3 can fish
100 g/ 1/3 cup tofu
1-2 eggs

Information from Canada's Food Guide

BODY MASS INDEX (BMI)

Make the most of the body type you have. For example, you can't be tall and willowy if your body shape is short and muscular. All the research agrees that any kind of dieting is out.

Now, let's check where you are on the Body Mass Index (BMI) chart.

Are you carrying some extra pounds?
Are they "weighing" you down? Robbing you of your energy?

In both Canada and the United States, weight loss has become a national obsession. In fact, at any given time, 56% of Canadian women are on diets and 70% of Canadian women want to lose weight. These statistics were taken from a study done by Health and Welfare Canada in 1991. These statistics are quite alarming and in even more recent studies the researchers have found that over half of the Canadian population is overweight.

So, how do we determine our "ideal body weight"? First of all we need to understand that our body consists of muscle, fat, water and bone. When we jump on the scale we must remember that all these variables exist. Over-fat is different from over-weight and muscles weigh more than fat because muscle tissue holds more water. Therefore, we must be careful in how we judge the results of the scale. At best, body weight gives only a rough estimate of body composition and therefore overall health. Most of us know when we are carrying too much weight. It literally slows us down and we are less energetic. It is more difficult to move, to walk up a flight of stairs, to get on the floor and play with our kids. More important, it is a health factor.

The most practical measurement used to determine our body weight, with relation to our level of health and therefore our level of energy, is the Body Mass Index (BMI). BMI is used to gauge an adult's risk for lifestyle diseases.

The BMI is designed for adults aged 20 to 65 years – those whose body size and composition are fairly stable.

It does not apply to babies, children, adolescents, pregnant or nursing women, senior citizens, very muscular people or endurance athletes such as runners.

Plot your current height and weight on this Chart:

- **Put an X at your height on Scale A**
- **Put an X at your weight on Scale B**
- **Using a ruler, draw a line to join the two X's**
- **Extend this line to Scale C**

Where the line meets on Scale C is your BMI.

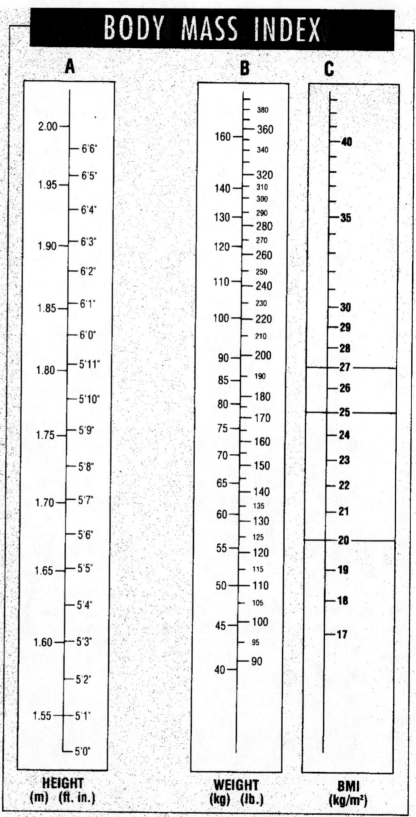

BODY MASS INDEX

Adapted from a chart produced by Health and Welfare Canada.

Now read through the chart below to discover where you sit in the health risk area.

BMI less than 20 A BMI of less than 20 may contribute to health problems in some people. Some of the health risks you face by being underweight are: ➢ **Heart irregularities** ➢ **Depression and other emotional distress** ➢ **Anemia**	**BMI 20–25** This is a good range for most people. If you fall within this zone and eat sensibly, your weight shouldn't cause any health problems.
BMI 25–27 This is a caution zone; watch your weight. While still within an acceptable range, a BMI of 25-27 could lead to health problems for some people.	**BMI greater than 27** The higher your BMI goes above 27, the more you risk developing these health problems: ➢ **High blood pressure** ➢ **Diabetes** ➢ **Heart disease** ➢ **Certain cancers**

Above information is from "Health, It's a Great Feeling", by the Ontario Ministry of Health

In June 1998, it was decided what a healthy weight would be utilizing the BMI. That number is 20-25. If you feel that you are at a health risk with your BMI number, please seriously consider taking action toward better health. In taking action you will decrease your risk of disease and increase your energy.

We can increase our body's metabolism by regularly making good food choices, drinking sufficient water and becoming more physically active. In fact our research states that the most direct way to increase your energy is to eat early, eat often, eat small amounts, reduce your overall fat intake, remain hydrated and include a small amount of protein and sufficient complex carbohydrates at every meal and snack.

Let's do it and become a more energetic you!

We need to gain knowledge and retrain our taste buds and learn to love less fattening foods.

My BMI is _____

> **Remember, making healthier food choices now is just as important to your future as having a sound financial plan.**
> *-Phyllis Reid-Jarvis*

CARBOHYDRATES ARE 100% PURE ENERGY

Carbohydrates are the stored form of energy found in plants and constitute the single most important energy source for humans. Keep in mind that proteins build and carbohydrates burn. Eat carbohydrates with a small amount of protein to gain the most benefit. That means choosing carbohydrates at every meal or snack. **Check your plate and look for about ¾ carbohydrates and only ¼ protein.**

Remember Carbohydrates are found in plant foods, are rich in starch and are packed with fibre, vitamins and minerals.

COMPLEX CARBOHYDRATES – include more nutrients and burn more slowly - keeping you ENERGIZED for longer periods. (28.4 grams = 1 ounce)

Grains: (each serving provides 15 grams of carbohydrates)
½ cup cooked - barley, bulgar, couscous, grits, kasha, millet, polenta
1 oz - cereals (¼ cup concentrated cereal, i.e. granola or grape nuts,
½-¾ cup flaked cereals, 1 cup puffed cereals)   1 slice – bread
5 crackers or mini rice cakes   2 crisp breads or rice cakes
½ cup uncooked – oats   1 fat free – tortilla
¼ cup – wheat germ
Vegetables: (each serving provides 15 grams of carbohydrates)
½ cup cooked – black eyed peas, green peas, corn, rutabagas, turnips, potatoes (white & sweet), winter squash, lima beans
Vegetables: (each serving provides 10 grams of carbohydrates)
½ cup cooked, 1 cup raw or 1 cup juiced – asparagus, beets, broccoli, Brussels sprouts, cabbage, carrots, cauliflower, celery, green beans, green leafy vegetables, kale, mushrooms, okra, onions, snow peas, sugar snaps, summer squash, tomatoes, zucchini
Fruits: (each serving provides 10 grams of carbohydrates)
½ fruit, ½ cup juice with pulp, ⅛ cup dried fruits – apples, apricots, berries, cherries, dates, grapefruit, grapes, kiwis, lemons, limes, melons, nectarines, oranges, peaches, pears, pineapples, plums and raisins

SIMPLE CARBOHYDRATES – include fewer nutrients and burn more quickly - giving you quick energy over a short period.

Simple carbohydrates are when we break down the carbohydrate to its simplest form, i.e. juice, sugars, honey, jams, jellies, syrups, candy, white flour, etc.

CARBOHYDRATE TIPS
- **Eat more <u>complex</u> carbohydrates throughout the day (introduce these slowly into your daily diet if you are not used to them).**
- **Choose bright, go for colour – brighter & deeper colour = more nutrients.**
- **Remember, ¾ of your plate complex carbohydrates and ¼ protein.**
- **Check your daily carbohydrate gram needs on page 34.**

ADD THESE "SUPER" CARBOHYDRATES

CHOOSE FOODS RICH IN
PHYTOCHEMICALS – ANTIOXIDANTS

The following fruits and vegetables are high in phytochemicals/antioxidants, include Vitamins C & E, and work to deactivate free radicals in our bodies. Free radicals change the LDL (bad) cholesterol so that it sticks to our artery walls. These unstable free radicals are also associated with cancer, heart disease and the effects of aging.

These free radical fighters are found in brightly coloured fruits and vegetables, adding beta-carotene, lycopene, lutein, and flavonoids.

Top Antioxidant Sources are:
Put a check beside those you will build into your daily diet.
(in alphabetical order)

Fruits	Vegetables
Apples (red)	**Beets**
Apricots, plums	**Broccoli**
Bananas	**Brussels Sprouts**
Blackberries	**Cabbage (red/green)**
Blueberries	**Carrots**
Cherries	**Corn**
Cranberries	**Garlic**
Dates	**Green Beans**
Grapes (red/green)	**Green Peppers**
Kiwis	**Lettuce**
Mangoes	**Onion**
Melon	**Peas**
Oranges	**Pumpkins**
Pineapple	**Red Pepper**
Pink grapefruit	**Spinach**
Prunes	**Squash**
Raisins	**Sweet Potatoes**
Raspberries	**Swiss Chard**
Strawberries	**Tomatoes**

* reprinted with permission from The Nutrition Action Health Letter, Copyright 2001 CSPI. Reprinted from National Action Health Letter (1875 Connecticut Ave., NW, Suite 300, Washington, DC 20009-5728). $36.00 Cdn.

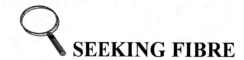 # SEEKING FIBRE

For a food to be considered a source of fibre it needs to contain at least 2g of fibre. A "good" source of fibre would have at least 4g per serving and a high fibre source would have 6g of fibre per serving.

We want 25 to 30 grams of fibre each day.

Lets think FIBRE and look over this list of items.
Number sequentially from 1 to 10 with #1 – LEAST up to #10 – MOST.

_____ **Pork and Beans, 1 cup**

_____ **Ovenjoy 100% Whole Wheat Bread, 2 slices**

_____ **Shreddies Cereal, ⅔ cup**

_____ **Triscuit Crackers, 4 crackers**

_____ **Chicken Noodle Soup, 1 cup**

_____ **Red River Cereal, hot, ¼ cup dry**

_____ **Primo Mixed Beans, ½ cup**

_____ **Minestrone Soup, 1 cup**

_____ **Wonder White Bread, 1 slice**

_____ **Bean and Bacon soup, 1 cup**

Read over the next page and learn more about Fibre before going to page 36 for the answers. Don't forget to Read Those Labels, page 40.

NOTES ON FIBRE

Fibre helps keep our bodies healthy and feeling full longer. We need 25-30 grams of fibre each day.

Fibre is the part of fruits, vegetables and grains that our body cannot digest. We need this fibre to help move the food we eat through our digestive system. In eating sufficient fibre we feel full and satisfied faster. Fibre can also help us to avoid overeating, keeping our weight in balance. Getting sufficient fibre also helps us avoid health problems such as; diabetes, heart attacks and strokes, digestive disorders, constipation, hemorrhoids, appendicitis, diverticulosis, impotency, cancer and weight gain. Carrying extra weight weighs us down, tires us out, and is an energy robber.

Make sure you get enough fibre.
Choose fewer refined carbohydrates like white flour, sugar, and white rice.
Choose MORE COMPLEX CARBOHYDRATES like:

WHOLE GRAIN
This means using whole-wheat flour, brown rice (triples your fibre), whole-wheat pasta, whole-wheat tortilla, whole-wheat crackers, whole oats, etc. We get fooled sometimes when the words 'wheat flour' are used (it's not necessarily whole wheat) or 'enriched bread' (this is when they take out about 21 nutrients in the refining process and add back about 4). Choose FLAX - ½ cup delivers 6 grams of fibre. Compare this with 1 ½ cups of cooked oatmeal for the same 6 grams.

Fresh FRUIT
Eat the peel too. Nibble on a few dried fruits. They are just as good as fresh.

Sprinkle ground flaxseed on your cereal, add some to your recipes.

Add those fresh VEGETABLES. Eating raw vegetables adds more fibre. Sneak them in whenever you can.

What about those BEANS?
Yes, they are full of complex carbohydrate fibre and protein.
Add beans to your day. Add a few to your soups and stews.
Have beans as your protein instead of meats a couple of times a week. Remember canned beans are just as good as fresh. *Try soaking fresh beans several hours or overnight before cooking, rinse away your soaking water and cook according to your recipe. Soaking cuts the gas/bloating problems.*

WATCH WATER WALK WEIGHTS WONDERFUL

WATCH –what you eat!

I choose to fill my plate with ¾ carbohydrates at every meal and snack.
I <u>look</u> for ways to increase my daily fibre intake.

My notes on Carbohydrates:

I can get more Carbohydrates and more Fibre into my meals and snacks throughout the day by:

Are you OVERLOADING your plate? Or, are you using a plate that is too large? Measure your food intake.
Place your hands together, palms up. The amount of food that will easily (not mounded, not overflowing) fit into your palms is a good indicator of the amount of food your body needs at any main meal. Remember your stomach is about the size of one and one half of your own fists.

FIND THE FAT EXERCISE

The intake of dietary fat is one of the critical factors in optimal health and weight management. We need fat for energy. But how much and what type of fat?

Let's think FAT. Look over this list of items.
Number sequentially from 1 to 9, with #1 – LEAST FAT up to #9 – MOST FAT.

_____ **One medium Egg**

_____ **One small Hot Dog Wiener**

_____ **One cup (250ml or 8oz) of Chocolate Milk**

_____ **One can of Sardines (128g or 4.5oz)**

_____ **One medium Rice Crispy Square**

_____ **Three slices of Light Klik Sandwich Meat**

_____ **One instant Oatmeal Porridge packet (plain)**

_____ **One Glazed Chocolate Cake Donut**

_____ **Soybean Snacking Nuts (40g or 1.4oz)**

Read over the next few pages and learn more about fat before going to page 37 for the answers.
Don't Forget to Read Those Labels, page 40.

FATS ARE A DIRECT SOURCE OF ENERGY

We need some fat in our diets. Fats provide energy. Fats cushion and insulate our body, store energy for times when we need it, transport those fat-soluble vitamins (A, D, E & K) throughout our bodies. Fats supply two essential fatty acids that the body can't make itself (Omega-3 and Omega-6). They also allow the gallbladder to function properly and help prevent gallstones, provide taste and texture to our foods, and help us to feel full and satisfied. Both Canadians and Americans are taking in more fat than we can burn and it is being stored as excess body fat. Too much fat can lead to high rates of heart disease, obesity, and cancer. It also can make us feel sluggish and exhausted. Too much fat weighs us down and tires us out. Somehow, we need to get just the right amount and the best type of fat to be at peak energy levels.

Let's learn a little more about the differences in fats to help us choose our source of fats wisely.

Saturated Fats: **Choose as little of these as possible.**

Primarily found in animal sources like fatty meats and chicken skin. Also from dairy products like whole milk, butter, cheeses, in egg yolks, lard and in tropical oils like palm kernel and coconut oil. These fats can raise our cholesterol levels.

Monounsaturated Fats: **Choose more of these.**

The highest amount is found in olives and olive oil, canola oil, avocados, most nuts, peanut oil, and sesame oil. Monounsaturated fat <u>may</u> help lower our LDL (low-density lipoproteins), the "bad" cholesterol.

Polyunsaturated Fats: **Choose more of these.**

Found in oils, grains, seeds, nuts, soy foods such as tofu and some vegetables. These fats are needed for fat storage, for cellular health, and <u>may</u> help us lower our LDL cholesterol levels. Polyunsaturated fats include the essential Omega-3 and Omega-6 fatty acids. Omega 3's are important for growth, reproduction, and vision – see the next page.

Hydrogenation - (Trans-Fats):   **Choose as little of these as possible.**

This is when we artificially pump hydrogen into fats and oils to stiffen them to make them more spreadable. This process changes their molecular structure from "cis" to "trans". We call them trans-fatty acids. Excessive use of hydrogenated oils can lead to health problems. Even partial hydrogenation may raise total cholesterol levels. Choose reduced fat, low or no hydrogenation soft tub margarine. Remember the harder the fat is at room temperature, the more harm it does to your arteries.

The latest research recommends we choose a low source of saturated fats, a good source of polyunsaturated fats and some monounsaturated fats. Here are the results of the August, 2002, Nutrition Action Health Letter's research on oils.

From the lowest in Saturated Fats on the left to the highest in Saturated Fats on the right.

Canola Oil (low in sats, good mix of poly & mono)	Cottonseed
Flaxseed Oil (most Omega-3's)	Chicken Fat
Safflower Oil	Lard (pork fat)
Sunflower Oil	Beef tallow
Corn Oil	Palm Oil
Olive Oil (most mono)	Butter
Sesame Oil	Cocoa Butter
Soybean Oil (low in sats, good mix poly & mono)	Palm Kernel Oil
Peanut Oil	Coconut Oil (highest is saturated fat)

Fats that we take in as straight dietary fats (oils, butter and margarine, cream) are most easily stored in our body as fat. It takes only 3 calories of energy expenditure to convert 100 calories of fat into new stored body fat. It takes eight times as many calories - 24 calories to turn 100 calories of complex carbohydrates into stored body fat. So you can see, fat stores as fat quite efficiently.

Be careful not to overeat when you see low fat or no fat options. Sometimes, when we choose "no-fat", we think we can eat as much as we want and it won't turn to stored body fat. But, if you are taking in more calories from fat, protein or carbohydrates than you burn off, your body will simply store them as body fat.

NOTE: *The fat in high fat foods causes mental and physical fatigue.*

OMEGA-3 AND OMEGA-6 ESSENTIAL FATTY ACIDS

These two essential fatty acids are important for growth, cell membranes, hormones, and nerve coverings. They keep our blood from becoming too sticky and forming clots, and they help lower Low Density Lipoproteins (LDL) and triglyceride levels. Our bodies don't manufacture Omega-3s or Omega-6s and so we must get them from the foods we eat.

We get sufficient Omega-6s more easily from our diet as they are found in vegetable oils, meat, fish, and eggs. So getting them is really not a concern. But, we don't seem to be getting enough Omega-3s.

Omega-3s can be found in polyunsaturated fats. Our best sources are Flaxseed Oil, Canola Oil, and Soybean Oil. The best source here is flaxseed oil with 2.5g in each teaspoon. So don't take more than ½ tsp. You can also sprinkle some ground flaxseed over your cereal or add it to your baking.

Health Canada recommends that we get between 1.2 and 1.6 grams (1,200 mg to 1,600 mg) of Omega-3 fatty acids every day.

But the U.S. Food and Drug Administration warn us that getting more than 3 grams (3,000 mg) of Omega-3 per day may raise a risk of hemorrhagic stroke.

Seafood Sources of Omega-3 Fatty Acids (6 oz. = 170g)

Perch - 6 oz.	0.7g	Oysters -3 oz.	1.1g
Halibut - 6 oz.	0.8g	Scallops - 6 oz.	0.6g
Flounder/Sole - 6 oz.	0.9g	Shrimp - 3 oz.	0.3g
Mackerel - 3oz.canned	1.0g	Lobster - 3 oz.	0.3g
Tuna, White - 3 oz.	0.7g	Crab - 3 oz.	0.4g
Cod, Pacific - 6 oz.	0.5g	Salmon, Atlantic - 6 oz.	3.7g
Herring, pickled - 3 oz.	1.2g	Snapper - 3 oz.	1.3g

If you are not eating fish two to three times each week, try taking a fish oil supplement to meet your Omega-3 needs. If you choose a supplement, look for about 1 gram per day.

FAT TIPS
- **Reduce your overall intake of fat. (all fats are 9 calories per gram)**
- **Spread your fat grams over the day, i.e. some at every meal and snack.**
- **Trim all visible fat from meats and remove the skin from poultry.**
- **Use only low or no-fat dairy products, dressings, cheeses, peanut butter, etc.**
- **Don't BINGE ON LOW FAT foods–they are often high in calories.**
- **Watch the types of fat you are choosing.**
- **Check YOUR daily FAT gram needs on page 35.**

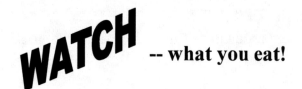

WATCH WATER WALK WEIGHTS WONDERFUL

WATCH -- what you eat!

I've cut down my intake of saturated fats.
I've increased my intake of polyunsaturated fats and Omega-3 fatty acids.
I choose "low or no" fat products

My notes on Fat:

I can reduce my daily Fat intake by:

I can increase my daily Omega-3 Fatty Acid intake by:

PROTEIN AS AN ENERGY BUILDER

Proteins are our body's building blocks – helping us build muscle tissue. Protein works to replace worn out cells, regulate our body functions, boost our metabolism, and stabilize our energy levels. Protein helps us stay full longer.

Protein is mainly found in anything that comes from an animal. Small amounts are also found in most plants, with a slightly larger amount found in the legume family. The legume pods absorb the nitrogen found in the soil and they become a good high fibre, low fat source of protein. Legumes are an incomplete protein, as they do not contain all the essential amino acids. They need to be combined with a grain or a seed product, i.e. peanut butter with whole wheat bread or beans with brown rice.

It is important to get sufficient quality protein throughout the day. We, as North Americans are consuming about five times more protein than our body needs. Therefore, we recommend that you have a *small* portion of quality protein at every meal and snack. An exception might be for body builders where they are constantly building and breaking down muscle tissue.

Main Protein Sources

Dairy Products, (like cheese, milk, yogurt)	Meat (make it lean)	Poultry
Fish, Sea Food	Peanut Butter	Egg Whites
Legumes/Beans Soybean Products		

ADD PROTEIN TO YOUR MEALS AND SNACKS THROUGH THE DAY
(each serving equals <u>7 grams of protein</u>)

- 6 oz. - no-fat milk or no-fat yogurt
- 1 oz. or ¼ cup grated - low fat cheeses
- ¼ cup - no-fat or 1% low-fat cottage cheese, part skim or fat free ricotta
- 1 – egg
- 1 oz. – flaked fish (tuna, salmon)
- ¼ cup - seafood (crab, lobster)
- 5 pieces – seafood (shrimp, oysters, scallops, clams)
- 1 oz. or ¼ cup – poultry
- 1 oz. – beef, pork, veal, lamb (choose lean - trim the fat)
- ¼ cup – legumes (beans – black, garbanzo, kidney, navy, red, great northern, soy, and lentils, split peas, other soy products like tofu, and soy milk)
- 1 tbsp. – natural peanut butter

Add skim milk powder to your recipes.

(adapted from "Energy Edge" by Pamela Smith, R.D.)

PROTEIN TIPS
- **Have small amounts of protein throughout the day.**
- **Choose lean protein.**
- **We need about 40-100 grams of protein each day.**
- **Check your daily protein gram needs on page 35.**

WATCH WATER WALK WEIGHTS WONDERFUL

WATCH --what you eat!

*I choose to add a <u>small</u> amount of protein at every meal and snack I eat
never more than ¼ of my plate.
I give my body sufficient protein to keep my body strong.*

My notes on Protein:

I can get small amounts of Protein at every snack and meal I eat throughout the day by:

CALORIE GRID AND INDIVIDUAL GRAM FORMULA

We do not recommend that you start counting calories and we are not in favor of dieting. We have, however, included this grid to enable you to get an idea of the numbers of calories and grams of carbohydrates, fats and proteins recommended for your calorie intake. Use the following table as a guideline only. Remember you need sufficient calories to give you energy. But if you take in more calories than you burn off - they will be stored as fat, no matter which food source they come from.

AN ESTIMATE OF MY PERSONAL CALORIE NEEDS

Choose a category that fits you.	Desired weight:	Multiply by:	Your Daily Calorie Limit
A sedentary woman	lbs.	X 12=	
A sedentary man	lbs.	X 14=	
A moderately active woman	lbs.	X 15=	
A moderately active man	lbs.	X 17=	
A very active woman	lbs.	X 18=	
A very active man	lbs.	X 20=	

My ESTIMATED OPTIMUM daily CALORIE intake requirement _____

CARBOHYDRATES
- Every gram of carbohydrates has 4 calories.
- Strive to get about 60% of your total daily calories from carbohydrates.
- We need between 60 to 360 grams of carbohydrates per day (depending on our size and activity level).
  To find out your personal carbohydrate gram needs, take your Optimum Calorie Intake above, times the 60% recommended, then divide by the number of calories in carbohydrates.
  _____Calories X .60=_____ ÷4 = _____grams per day.

FAT
- Every gram of fat has 9 calories no matter what type of fat it is.
- Strive to get about 20% to 30% of your total daily calories from fats.
- Remember you only want 10% to 15% of these fat grams to be from saturated fat.
  To find out your personal fat gram needs, take your Optimum Calorie Intake above, times 30%, then divide by the number of calories in fat.
  _____Calories X .30 =_____ ÷ 9 =_____grams per day.

PROTEIN
- Every gram of protein has 4 calories.
- Strive to get about 15% of your total daily calories from proteins.
- We need about 40 to 100 grams (4 to 6 oz. or the size of a deck of cards) of protein each day.
  To find out your personal protein gram needs, take your Optimum Calorie Intake above, times the 15% recommended, then divide by the number of calories in protein.
  _____Calories X .15 =_____ ÷ 4 =_____grams per day.

(adapted from "Low Fat Living" by Cooper & Cooper, and "Picture Perfect Weight Loss" by Dr. Shapiro)

ANSWER SHEET – SEEKING FIBRE

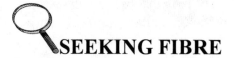

SEEKING FIBRE

For a food to be considered a source of fibre it needs to contain at least 2 grams of fibre. A "good" source of fibre would have at least 4 grams per serving and a high fibre source would have 6 grams of fibre per serving.

Yes!   We want 25 to 30 grams of fibre each day.

Number from 1 to 10, with #1 – LEAST FIBRE up to #10 – MOST FIBRE.

No. & Grams of Fibre

1 - (0g)   Wonder White Bread, 2 slices

2 - (0.3g)   Chicken Noodle Soup, 1 cup

3 - (2g)   Triscuit Crackers, 4 crackers

4 - (3g)   Shreddies Cereal, 2/3 cup

5 - (4.5g)   Primo Mixed Beans, ½ cup

5 - (4.5g)   Minestrone Soup, 1 cup

6 - (5g)   Ovenjoy 100% Whole Wheat Bread, 2 slices

7 - (5.79g)   Red River Cereal, hot, ¼ cup dry

8 - (12g)   Pork and Beans, 1 cup

9 - (14.6g)   Bean and Bacon soup, 1 cup

So! How did you do?

Remember to 'Read Those Labels', page 40.

ANSWER SHEET - FIND THE FAT EXERCISE

Choose fat that builds energy and doesn't weigh you down. Remember we need fat in our diets. However, we want to cut our saturated fats to only 10% to 15% of our total daily fat gram intake. So you want to spend your Saturated Fat grams wisely.

Remember #1 has the LEAST FAT up to #9 with the MOST FAT

__1__   ONE INSTANT OATMEAL PORRIDGE PACKET
2 grams of Fat – low to no Saturated Fat
This is a good choice, especially if you add only Skim Milk. This packet contains Thiamin, Niacin, Vitamin B6, Folacin, Pantoghenic, Acid, and Iron.
*4.6g Protein
*36g Carbohydrates (3.1g Fibre)

__1__   ONE RICE CRISPY SQUARE -   2 grams of Fat
Low in Fat and also has some Vitamin D, Vitamin B2, Niacin, Folacin, and Iron.
*.7g Protein
*18g Carbohydrates (.1g Fibre)

__2__   ONE CUP (8 oz/250g) **CHOLOLATE MILK -   4-5 grams of Saturated Fat**
Watch the LABELS be sure of your quantity. Choose the 1% BF for the lower grams of Saturated Fat. This one is not a bad choice as it contains Vitamins A, D, and Calcium.
*4.3g Protein
*12g Carbohydrates

__3__   ONE MEDIUM EGG -   5 grams of Saturated Fat
Yes an egg has 5 grams of Saturated Fat in the yolk. But look at the nutritional value this 5 grams of Saturated Fat brings – Vitamins A, D & E, Thiamin, Riboflavin, Niacin, Vitamins B6 & B12, Folacin, Pantothenic Acid, Calcium, Phosphorus, Magnesium, Iron and Zinc. Wow! Note: **Add some whole wheat bread and turn this one into an energy star*.**
6g of Protein
0.5g of Carbohydrates

__4__   ONE CAN OF SARDINES - **8 grams of Fat –BUT only 1.8 of these are Saturated.**
Here is an excellent choice to help us get the Fats that our bodies need the most – Omega-3 (1.2g), Omega-6 (.2g), Monounsaturated (4g), Polyunsaturated (2g). This choice also has Calcium and Iron. Note: **Add some whole wheat crackers or whole wheat bread and make this into an energy star*.**
19 g Protein
0 g Carbohydrates

5   **ONE SMALL HOT DOG WIENER -**   8.5 grams of Saturated Fat
*For this choice of Saturated Fat you are getting very little nutritional value.
And – are you really only going to eat one?*
? Low Protein
0 Carbohydrates

6   **THREE SLICES OF LIGHT KLIK LUNCHEON MEAT –**
11 grams of Saturated Fat   *Very little nutritional value here.*
Some Protein
0 Carbohydrates

7   **40 GRAMS OF SOYBEAN SNACKING NUTS –**
12 grams of Fat – BUT only 1.5g of Saturated Fat.
*This snack does have a high Fat content BUT it is mostly the Fat we need
and want. Here we do get the Fats that are good for us, i.e. 5.5g of
Polyunsaturated Fat and 4.8g of Monounsaturated Fat.*
*14g Protein
*9.7g Carbohydrates (3.9g Fibre)

8   **ONE GLAZED CHOCOLATE CAKE DONUT -**
22 grams of mostly Saturated Fat.
Here we have mostly Saturated Fat and very little nutritional value.
? Protein, some from the eggs and milk content
**? Carbohydrates – mostly refined carbohydrates – so would be a "quick
burn".**

All the above show us that we must 'Read Those Labels' and think about our food choices. To maintain our energy we want to choose snacks and meals that have both carbohydrates and proteins.

Go back over the last two pages and find the   *   for our energy building "star" snacks.

For a sustained level of energy we want to choose complex carbohydrates and the best have some degree of fibre content. Complex Carbohydrates move more slowly through our systems, keeping us feeling full longer and sustaining our energy levels over longer periods of time.

CHOOSE FROM THIS LIST OF ENERGIZING SNACKS

Before you even have a snack, check that you aren't just thirsty.

> **Drink a wonderful
> glass of cool water.**

Also, check your hunger level. If you still feel real hunger then choose one of these energizing snacks.

Watch the number of calories and type of fat in your snack choices.

Some snack ideas containing both carbohydrates and proteins are:

- **a glass of orange juice, 1 tbsp. peanut butter on 2 whole wheat crackers**
- **rice cakes with natural peanut butter**
- **fresh fruit or small box of raisins and low-fat cheese**
- **half a lean turkey or chicken sandwich on whole wheat bread**
- **plain, nonfat yogurt blended with any fruit or all fruit jam**
- **whole grain cereal with skim milk**
- **baked low fat tortilla chips with fat-free bean dip and salsa**
- **popcorn sprinkled with parmesan cheese**
- **crisp bread with sliced turkey and Dijon mustard**
- **small pop-top can of water-packed tuna or chicken, with whole grain crackers**
- **whole grain crackers or raisin squares cereal and low-fat cheese half of a small whole wheat bagel or English muffin with 1 tbsp. light cream cheese**
- **fruit shake--skim milk blended with frozen fruit and vanilla flavoring**
- **a packet of instant oatmeal porridge with a bit of skim milk**
- **homemade low-fat bran muffin with low-fat or skim milk**
- **dried fruit of any kind along with a few nuts like walnuts, pecans, sunflower seeds and raisins – package into ¼ cup baggies**

(adapted in part from "The Energy Edge" by Pamela Smith. R.D.)

Reminder:

> Snacks work great for keeping your energy constant throughout the day. But, if you add snacks and don't cut down on your meal size – you could be taking in too many calories.

READ THOSE LABELS

You have been reading about making good food and drink choices that help you maintain your health and energy levels. A big part of making good choices is to watch what you put into your mouth. Remember "We Are What We Eat". In making these choices we need to stop and read the labels.

Canada has recently (January, 2003) improved the requirements for food labeling to better reflect the nutritional content of the packaged contents. So the next time you reach for anything off the grocery shelf – read it carefully and make the "best" choices.

They should look something like this.

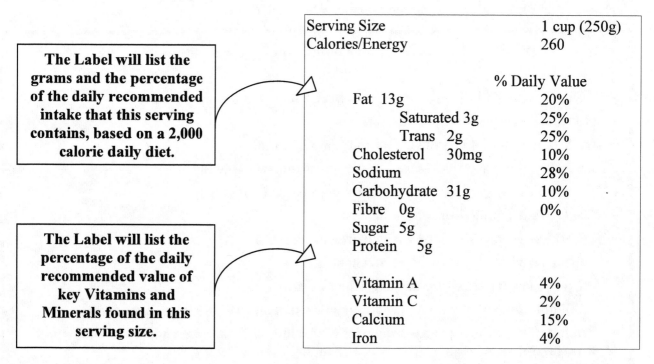

Serving Size	1 cup (250g)
Calories/Energy	260

	% Daily Value
Fat 13g	20%
Saturated 3g	25%
Trans 2g	25%
Cholesterol 30mg	10%
Sodium	28%
Carbohydrate 31g	10%
Fibre 0g	0%
Sugar 5g	
Protein 5g	
Vitamin A	4%
Vitamin C	2%
Calcium	15%
Iron	4%

The Label will list the grams and the percentage of the daily recommended intake that this serving contains, based on a 2,000 calorie daily diet.

The Label will list the percentage of the daily recommended value of key Vitamins and Minerals found in this serving size.

What is important is that you 'Read those Labels'.

Decide if the serving size that the information is based on is indeed the portion size that you will be eating. You may have larger portions and that means you must double or triple the listed quantities. It is difficult for us sometimes to compare foods as they tend to use different portion sizes. So be careful.

Ask yourself these questions:
- Do I have my eating plan in mind and my shopping list written and in my pocket?
- Does this food fit for my building energy food choices?
- Is it an energy gain or an energy drain?
- Does the serving size listed reflect the amount I will actually eat?

VITAMIN AND MINERAL SUPPLEMENTS

Vital nutrients are required to burn stored fat, turning those calories into energy. These vital nutrients are the vitamins and minerals in our foods and in the supplements we may choose to add to our daily personal health care.

TO TAKE OR NOT TO TAKE?   WHAT TO TAKE?
HOW MUCH TO TAKE?   WHEN TO TAKE?

We all know that it is best to get our vitamins and minerals through our daily food choices as there are complex combinations between our foods that maximize the benefit to our body. But, do we remain so nutritionally correct that we get all the vitamins and minerals we need every day? In fact, as we age, our bodies' even stop producing some of these needed vitamins and minerals.

Our research supports taking a good multi-vitamin with minerals once each day with a meal.

Before beginning a vitamin supplement, check with your doctor. Some supplements may interfere with medications that you are taking. Listen to your body. Talk to your pharmacist – they can bring a wealth of knowledge. Read over the NEW NAS (National Academy of Sciences) recommended intake on the next two pages and compare it with any vitamin supplement you decide to take. We want and need the right amount of each and every vitamin and mineral we require to be at our healthiest and energetic best.

Never use cola, tea, or coffee to take your vitamins as they contain tannic acid and interfere with the absorption of iron. Drink wonderful water instead.

The next two pages are reproduced research from the *Nutrition Action Health Letter, National Academy of Sciences, June 2001.

So check your daily food intake against the amount of each vitamin and mineral you need every day. Are you getting them regularly from food alone? If not, consider adding a daily multi-vitamin to your health care. When you are choosing a multi-vitamin check that
- they meet your special needs as to age and sex
- the amounts listed are within the guidelines of the RDI or the NAS recommendations
- all the vitamins and minerals are included
- the expiration date is several months away

1 gram (g) = 1,000 milligrams (mg) = 100,000 micrograms (mcg)

*the next two pages are reprinted with permission from The Nutrition Action <u>Health Letter, June, 2001</u>. Copyright <u>2001</u> CSPI. Reprinted from Nutrition Action Health Letter (1875 Connecticut Ave., NW, Suite 300, Washington DC 20009-5728). $36.00 Cnd.

VITAMINS

Nutrient (other names)	New NAS Recommended Intake	Recommended Daily Intake (RDI)	Good Sources	Upper Level (UL)	Selected Adverse Effects	Nutrition Action Comments
Vitamin A (retinol)	Women: 700 mcg Men: 900 mcg	3,330 IU[1] (1,000 RE or 1,000 mcg)	Liver, fatty fish, fortified foods (milk, margarine, etc.).	10,000 IU (3,000 mcg)	*Liver toxicity, birth defects.* Inconclusive: bone loss.	The body turns some carotenoids into vitamin A.
Carotenoids (alpha-carotene, beta-carotene, beta-cryptoxanthin, lutein, lycopene, zeaxanthin)	None. (NAS advises eating more cartotenoid-rich fruits and vegetables).	None	Orange fruits & vegetables (alpha- and beta-carotene), green leafy vegetables (beta-carotene and lutein), tomatoes (lycopene).	None. Panel said don't take beta-carotene, except to get RDI for vitamin A.	Smokers who took high doses of beta-carotene supplements (33,000-50,000 IU a day) had higher risk of lung cancer.	Lutein may lower risk of cataracts and degeneration of the retina. Lycopene may lower risk of prostate cancer.
Thiamin (vitamin B-1)	Women: 1.1 mg Men: 1.2 mg	1.3 mg	Breads, cereals, pasta, & foods made with "enriched" or whole-grain flour; pork.	None	None reported.	
Riboflavin (vitamin B-2)	Women: 1.1 mg Men: 1.3 mg	1.6 mg	Milk, yogurt, foods made with "enriched" or whole-grain flour.	None	None reported.	May lower risk of cataracts.
Niacin (vitamin B-3)	Women: 14 mg Men: 16 mg	23 mg (23 NE)	Meat, poultry, seafood, foods made with "enriched" or whole-grain flour.	35 mg[2]	*Flushing (burning, tingling, itching, redness),* liver damage.	Cholesterol-lowering doses of niacin should only be taken under a doctor's supervision.
Vitamin B-6 (pyridoxine)	Ages 19-50: 1.3 mg Women 50+: 1.5 mg Men 50+: 1.7 mg	1.8 mg	Meat, poultry, seafood, fortified foods (cereals, etc.), liver.	100 mg	*Reversible nerve damage (burning, shooting, tingling pains, numbness, etc.).*	May lower risk of heart disease (by lowering homocysteine levels).
Vitamin B-12 (cobalamin)	2.4 mcg	2 mcg	Meat, poultry, seafood, dairy foods, fortified foods (some veggie burgers and soy milks, etc.).	None	None reported.	People over 50 need a supplement or fortified food.
Folate (folacin, folic acid)	400 mcg	220 mcg (0.2 mg)	Orange juice, beans, other fruits & vegetables, fortified cereals, foods made with "enriched" or whole-grain flour.	1,000 mcg[2] (1 mg)	*Can mask or precipitate a B-12 deficiency, which can cause irreversible nerve damage.*	Reduces risk of birth defects. May lower risk of heart disease, cervical and colon cancer, and depression.
Vitamin C (ascorbic acid)	Women: 75 mg Men: 90 mg (Smokers: add 35 mg)	60 mg	Citrus & other fruits, vegetables, fortified juices.	2,000 mg	*Diarrhea.*	High doses (1,000 mg a day) may shorten colds.
Vitamin D	Ages 19-50: 200 IU[3] Ages 51-70: 400 IU[3] Over 70: 600 IU[3]	200 IU (5 mcg)	Sunlight, fatty fish, fortified foods (milk, liquid meal replacements like Ensure, etc.).	2,000 IU	*High blood calcium,* which may cause kidney and heart damage.	Deficiency can cause bone loss and may raise risk of osteoporosis.
Vitamin E (alpha-tocopherol)	15 mg (33 IU—synthetic) (22 IU—natural)	15 IU (synthetic)	Oils, whole grains, nuts.	1,000 mg[2] (1,100 IU—synthetic) (1,500 IU—natural)	*Hemorrhage.*	May lower risk of heart disease, prostate cancer, cataracts; may slow Alzheimer's.
Vitamin K (phylloquinone)	Women: 90 mcg[3] Men: 120 mcg[3]	80 mcg[4]	Green leafy vegetables, oils.	None	Interferes with coumadin & other anti-clotting drugs.	May lower risk of bone fractures.

Reproduced with permission from The Nutrition Action Health Letter, June 2001.

MINERALS

Nutrient (other names)	New NAS Recommended Intake	Recommended Daily Intake (RDI)	Good Sources	Upper Level (UL)	Selected Adverse Effects	Nutrition Action Comments
Calcium	Ages 19-50: 1,000 mg[3] Over 50: 1,200 mg[3]	1,100 mg	Dairy foods, leafy green vegetables, canned fish (eaten with bones).	2,500 mg	*High blood calcium,* which may cause kidney damage, kidney stones.	May lower risk of osteoporosis, colon cancer. High doses (2,000 mg a day) may raise risk of prostate cancer.
Chromium	Women: 20-25 mcg[3] Men: 30-35 mcg[3]	120 mcg[4]	Whole grains, bran cereals, meat, poultry, seafood.	None	Inconclusive: kidney or muscle damage.	May lower risk of diabetes.
Copper	900 mcg	2 mg[4] (2,000 mcg)	Liver, seafood, nuts, seeds, wheat bran, whole grains, chocolate.	10 mg (10,000 mcg)	*Liver damage.*	
Iron	Women 19-50: 18 mg Women 50+: 8 mg Men: 8 mg	14 mg	Red meat, poultry, seafood, foods made with "enriched" or whole-grain flour.	45 mg	*Gastrointestinal effects (constipation, nausea, diarrhea).*	Gene raises risk of iron overload (hemochromatosis) in some people.
Magnesium	Women: 310-320 mg Men: 400-420 mg	250 mg	Green leafy vegetables; whole-grain breads, cereals, etc.; nuts.	350 mg[2]	*Diarrhea.*	May lower risk of osteoporosis, heart disease, or high blood pressure.
Phosphorus	700 mg	1,100 mg	Dairy foods, meat, poultry, seafood, foods (processed cheese, colas, etc.) made with phosphate additives.	Ages 19-70: 4,000 mg Over 70: 3,000 mg	*High blood phosphorus,* which may damage kidneys and bones.	With phosphate additives on the rise, look for low-, not high-phosphorus multivitamins.
Selenium	55 mcg	70 mcg[4]	Seafood, meat, poultry; grains (depends on levels in soil).	400 mcg	Nail or hair loss or brittleness.	May lower risk of prostate, lung, colon cancer.
Zinc	Women: 8 mg Men: 11 mg	9 mg	Red meat, seafood, whole grains, fortified foods (breakfast cereals, liquid meal replacements, etc.).	40 mg	*Lower copper levels, HDL ("good") cholesterol, and immune response.*	The average person gets about a quarter of the UL from food.

New NAS Recommended Intake: Canada has not yet adopted these numbers, which come from the U.S. National Academy of Sciences (NAS) in collaboration with Canadian scientists. We list numbers for adults only.

Recommended Daily Intake (RDI): Unlike the new NAS recommended intakes, there is only one RDI for everyone over age two.

Tolerable Upper Intake Level (UL): These levels are upper safe daily limits. We list ULs for adults only.

Adverse Effects: What happens if you take too much. *The UL is based on the adverse effect listed in italics.* "Inconclusive" adverse effects are based on inconsistent or sketchy evidence.

Other Tolerable Upper Intake Levels

Boron: 20 mg	Manganese: 11 mg
Choline: 3.5 grams	Molybdenum: 2,000 mcg (2 mg)
Flouride: 10 mg	Nickel: 1 mg
Iodine: 1,100 mcg (1.1 mg)	Vanadium: 1.8 mg

[1] We get vitamin A both from retinol and carotenoids, but this number assumes that all of the vitamin A comes from retinol.

[2] From supplements and fortified foods only.

[3] Adequate Intake (AI). The NAS has too little data to set a recommended intake.

[4] U.S. Daily Value. No RDI has been set by Health Canada.

Reproduced with permission from The Nutrition Action Health Letter, June 2001.

QUALITY FOOD SOURCES OF VITAMINS AND MINERALS

(adapted in part from the University of California, Berkeley Wellness Letter)

POTASSIUM (Aim for about 3,500 mg a day, the US DV) Number of milligrams found in:
- *Beet greens, chopped, cooked – 1 cup = 1300*
- *Avocado – 6 oz = 1080*
- *Apricots, dried – ½ cup=895*
- *Beans (legumes), cooked 1 cup = 500-1200*
- *Potato, baked, with skin – 6oz = 710*
- *Clams, cooked – 3 oz = 535*
- *Yogurt, plain, low-fat 1 cup = 550*
- *Fish, most varieties, cooked – 4 oz = 350-700*
- *Orange Juice, fresh – 1 cup = 500*
- *Banana – 1 medium = 470*

VITAMIN C (RDI is 60 mg, but the Berkeley Wellness Letter recommended 250-500 mg). Number of milligrams found in:
- *Red Peppers – 4 oz = 215*
- *Orange juice, fresh – 1 c = 125*
- *Broccoli, chopped, cooked – 1 cup = 115*
- *Apple juice, with vitamin C – 1 cup = 105*
- *Green peppers – 4 oz = 100*
- *Brussels sprouts, cooked – 1cup = 95*
- *Grapefruit juice – 1 cup = 95*
- *Cranberry juice cocktail – 1 cup = 90*
- *Papaya – 5 oz = 90*
- *Strawberries, fresh – 1 cup = 85*

MAGNESIUM (RDI is 250mg) Number of milligrams found in:
- *Almonds/Hazelnuts – 2 oz = 170*
- *Spinach, fresh, cooked – 1 cup = 155*
- *Swiss Chard, fresh, cooked – 1 cup = 150*
- *Sunflower seeds, dried – ¼ cup = 130*
- *Halibut/Mackerel, cooked – 4 oz = 120*
- *Tofu – 4 oz = 120*
- *Wheat Bran – ¼ cup = 90*
- *Rice, brown, cooked – 1 cup = 85*
- *Avocado – 6 oz = 70*
- *Beans (legumes), cooked – 1 cup = 35*

FOLACIN (RDI is 220mcg) Number of micrograms found in:
- *Beans (legumes), cooked – 1 cup = 160-350*
- *Spinach, fresh, cooked – 1 cup = 260*
- *Oatmeal, fortified, instant – 1 cup = 200*
- *Asparagus, fresh, cooked – 6 spears = 130*
- *Avocado – 6 oz = 115*
- *Peas, green – 1 cup = 115*
- *Peas, green cooked – 1 cup = 95*
- *Brussels Sprouts, cooked – 1 cup = 95*
- *Wheat Germ – ¼ cup = 80*
- *Broccoli, chopped, cooked – 1 cup = 80*
- *Corn, Kernels – 1 cup = 75*

BETA CAROTENE (RDI-none listed) Number of milligrams found in:

- *Sweet Potatoes, cooked – 6 oz = 15*
- *Collard Greens, chopped, cooked 1 cup = 7*
- *Carrots – 1 medium = 5*
- *Cantaloupe – 6 oz = 5*
- *Squash, winter – 1 cup = 5*
- *Apricots, fresh – 3 medium = 4*
- *Pumpkin, fresh – 1 cup = 4*
- *Kale, cooked – 1 cup = 3*
- *Spinach, fresh, cooked – 1 cup = 3*
- *Mango, sliced – 1 cup = 2*

ZINC (RDI is 9mg) Number of milligrams found in:

- *Oysters, eastern – 3 oz = 150*
- *Crab, king – 4 oz = 9*
- *Beef, cooked – 4 oz = 6*
- *Wheat Germ – ¼ cup = 4*
- *Turkey, cooked – 4 oz = 4*
- *Lamb, cooked – 4 oz = 4*
- *Pork, cooked – 4 oz = 3*
- *Cashews/Almonds – 2 oz = 3*
- *Beans (legumes), cooked – 1 cup = 3*
- *Chicken, cooked – 4 oz = 2*

SELENIUM (RDI is 70mcg) Number of micrograms found in:

- *Brazil Nuts, dried – 1 oz = 840*
- *Tuna, canned – 4 oz = 80*
- *Oysters, cooked – 4oz = 80*
- *Flounder/Sole, cooked – 4 oz = 65*
- *Turkey, cooked – 4 oz = 40*
- *Chicken, cooked – 4 oz = 35*
- *Wheat Germ – ½ cup = 23*
- *Brown Rice, cooked, 1 cup = 20*
- *Oatmeal, cooked – 1 cup =19*
- *Egg, 1 medium = 14*

FIBRE (RDI=20-30grams) Number of grams found in:

- *Beans (legumes), cooked – 1 cup = 10-15*
- *Peas, green, cooked – 1 cup = 9*
- *Raspberries – 1 cup = 8*
- *Bulgur, cooked – 1 cup = 8*
- *Rye Wafers – 3 crackers = 7*
- *Wheat Bran – ¼ cup = 6*
- *Pasta, whole-wheat, cooked – 1 cup = 6*
- *Oat Bran, cooked – 1 cup = 6*
- *Squash, acorn – 4 oz = 5*
- *Potato, baked, with skin – 1 medium = 5*

1 gram (g) = 1,000 milligrams (mg) = 100,000 micrograms (mcg)

*Note: Your body can only absorb 500 mg of Calcium at one time.

CALCIUM* (see the age group requirements – we all may need an additional supplement here)
Number of milligrams found in:
- *Sour Cream, nonfat – 1 cup = 450*
- *Yogurt, plain, low-fat or nonfat – 1 cup = 435*
- *Sardines, canned, with bones – 4 oz = 430*
- *Collard greens, frozen, cooked – 1 cup = 360*
- *Ricotta Cheese, part-skim- ½ cup = 340*
- *Parmesan Cheese – 1 oz = 335*
- *Yogurt, low-fat fruit – 1 cup = 315*
- *Milk – 1 cup = 300*
- *Swiss Cheese – 1 oz = 270*
- *Salmon, canned, with bones – 4 oz = 260*
- *Orange Juice – Calcium Fortified – 1 cup = 364*

VITAMIN B6 (RDI is 1.8 mg). Number of milligrams found in:
- *Tuna, fresh, cooked - 4 oz = 1.2*
- *Potato, baked, with skin – 6 oz = 0.7*
- *Banana – 1 medium = 0.7*
- *Salmon, fresh, cooked – 4 oz = 0.7*
- *Chicken or turkey, cooked - 4 oz = 0.6*
- *Prune juice, canned – 1 cup = 0.6*
- *Pork, cooked – 4 oz = 0.6*
- *Avocado – 6 oz = 0.5*
- *Beef, cooked 4 oz = 0.5*
- *Sweet potato, cooked – 6 oz = 0.4*

VITAMIN B-12 (RDI is 2 mcg). Number of micrograms found in:
- *Clams - 3 oz = 84.0*
- *Atlantic Mackerel - 3 oz = 16.0*
- *Beef - 3oz = 3.0*
- *Tuna or Salmon – 3 = 2.0*
- *Milk – 8 oz = 1.5*

HEALTHY FOODS

These are the BEST foods based on their content of the Daily Recommended Value (RDI). They are listed in descending order. The "best" are first.

Based on: calories, carotenoids, vitamin C, folacin, potassium, fibre	Based on: carotenoids, vitamin C, folacin, potassium, calcium, iron, fibre	Based on: fibre, folic acid, magnesium, iron copper, zinc, protein	Based on: fibre, magnesium, B-6, zinc, copper, iron
## Fruit	## Vegetables ½ cup fresh, cooked, unless noted	## Beans 1 cup cooked	## Grains Includes Pasta & Potato for comparison 5 oz, cooked
1 Guava 2 c. Watermelon ½ Grapefruit, pink or red ½ med. or 1 c. cubed. Papaya 2 Kiwifruit ¼ Cantaloupe ½ c. Apricots, dried 1 Orange 8 Strawberries 4 Apricots 1 c. Blackberries ¼ c. Peaches, dried 1 c. Raspberries ½ Grapefruit, white 1 Tangerine 1 Persimmon ½ Mango 1/10 Honeydew Melon 1 Star Fruit - (Carambola) ½ c. Apricots canned 1 Lemon 1 Banana	Collard Greens, frozen Spinach Kale 1 med. Sweet Potato, no skin Swiss Chard ½ med. Red Pepper, raw Pumpkin, canned Carrots Broccoli 1 med. Carrot, raw, Okra Lettuce, cos or 1 c. romaine, raw Brussels Sprouts 1 c. Spinach, raw 1 Potato, baked with skin Squash, winter Mixed Vegetables, frozen ½ med. Green Pepper, raw Asparagus	Soybeans Pinto Beans Chickpeas – (garbanzos, ceci) Lentils Cranberry Beans Black-eyed Peas - cowpeas) Pink Beans Navy Beans Black Beans (turtle beans) Small White Beans White Beans Lima Beans, baby Kidney Beans, all types Adzuki Beans Great Northern Beans Mung Beans Lima Beans, large Broad Beans (fava beans) Peas, split (green) 4 oz. Tofu, raw	Potato, with skin Quinoa Macaroni or Spaghetti if whole wheat Amaranth Buckwheat groats Spaghetti, spinach Bulgar Barley, pearled Wild Rice Millet Brown Rice Triticale Spaghetti Wheat Berries Macaroni Kamut Oats, rolled Spelt White Rice, converted Couscous White Rice, instant Soba Noodles Corn Grits

* Reprinted with permission from The Nutrition Action Health Letter, June, 2001. Copyright 2001 CSPI. Reprinted from Nutrition Action Health Letter (1875 Connecticut Ave., NW, Suite 300, Washington DC 20009-5728). $36.00 Cdn.

WATER AS A SOURCE OF ENERGY

Dehydration is the number one cause of fatigue.
Without food, a person can survive for days, maybe even months –
BUT without water, we can survive for only three to five days.

Four elements our bodies must have to survive are: Oxygen, Water, Salt, and Potassium.

We all know we "should" drink 6 – 8 glasses of water every day. Now lets look at why this is so very important to our bodies, to our good health and our energy levels.

Our bodies are made up of about 70 thousand billion cells. Ask yourself the following questions:

How do we get the food to all these individual cells?

How do we break down the complicated lumps into tiny basic bits that the cell can absorb?

How do we take away the waste products of metabolism?

How do we get oxygen to each cell?

How do we get rid of the carbon dioxide produced?

How do we keep the temperature of this complex mass constant?

How do we grow, starting from one fertilized cell and ending up with 70 thousand billion cells?

How do we repair damaged cells and replace worn-out ones?

The answer to all of these questions is WATER, good clean water.

Water is the main component of all living, active cells. It is the essential substance in which all the metabolic activities of the cell occur and it is the matrix for the structural components of the cell. It is often referred to as the "universal solvent" (only slightly exaggerated) and its ability to ionize many of the substances it dissolves is crucial to a wide range of metabolic processes.

WATER
- **carries the enzymes and acid to break down the fats, proteins and carbohydrates**
- **is the essential element in digestion (hydrolysis means adding water)**
- **transports the tiny particles of digestion to every single cell through 60 miles (96 kilometres) of tubing**
- **removes carbon dioxide**
- **keeps the body's temperature constant**
- **allows the body to grow to adult size and to repair itself constantly as it breaks down**

There are 80 pounds of water in a 169-pound man and 6 pounds of water in an 8-pound baby.

If we don't keep our body well hydrated our body will react by
- increasing our fat deposits as our liver metabolizes less fat and more fat is stored
- poor kidney function
- retaining water as a lack of water is seen as a threat to survival
- exhibiting dehydration through, headaches, backaches and general fatigue

Drinking enough water can help our bodies to
- digest our food
- get rid of excess fluid
- use more fat as fuel because the liver is free to metabolize stored fat
- transport energizing nutrients throughout our bodies
- maintain proper muscle tone
- keep our skin healthy, resilient and wrinkle resistant
- get rid of waste
- relieve constipation
- lubricate our joints and provide a cushion helping our joints bear the force produced by weight or tension by muscle action on our joints
- regain our natural thirst
- stop eating when really we are thirsty

Increase your daily water intake gradually to about:
1 glass of water before each meal
little or no water with your meal
2 glasses mid-morning
2 glasses mid afternoon
(cool water is absorbed into your system more quickly)
Remember: Drink more when you exercise and when you drink fluids that dehydrate your body, i.e. containing caffeine or alcohol.

The majority of our research stated that water is the best way to hydrate our bodies. A few resources also counted fruit juice, skim milk, decaffeinated soda, tea and coffee. We suggest you drink these with your meal and continue your water intake.

Some symptoms of dehydration are: water retention, headaches, irritability, fatigue, chills, and dry skin, dry eyes and/or dry nose.
An easy way to check that you are getting sufficient water is to check the colour of your urine. The lighter -- the better.

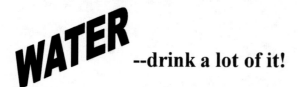

WATCH WATER WALK WEIGHTS WONDERFUL

WATER --drink a lot of it!

My skin and my body are well hydrated.
I drink eight glasses of water spread out over my day.

My notes on Water:

I can ensure that I drink at least six glasses of Water every day by:

BUILDING ENERGY THROUGH FOOD & WATER

It all boils down to making smart choices, over and over again. The healthier you can maintain your body through smart food choices, physical activity and restful sleep, the more energized you will be.

Our research supports that an energizing eating program includes three <u>smaller</u> meals and two to three <u>light</u> snacks each day. Start with breakfast (still the most critically important meal of the day), a mid-morning energizing snack, a small lunch, your afternoon pick me up, a light but full supper, and only if you are still hungry, a snack before bed. Remember to balance your plate *(a medium sized dinner plate)* with ¾ carbohydrates, ¼ proteins with a bit of fat spread throughout the day.

**Do not take in more calories than you burn. Eat slowly, pay attention and stop overeating.
Listen to your body.
It takes 20 to 30 minutes for your stomach to tell your brain that you are full.**

Your day could look like this:

1 glass of WATER on rising

<u>BREAKFAST</u>   complete with carbohydrates, proteins and a small amount of fat

2 glasses of WATER during the morning
(remember cold water is absorbed more quickly)

Mid-Morning Snack - carbohydrates and proteins

1 glass of WATER before lunch

<u>LUNCH</u>   complete with carbohydrates, proteins and a small amount of fat

2 glasses of WATER during the afternoon

Mid Afternoon Snack - carbohydrates and proteins

1 glass of WATER before supper

> *Avoid drinking caffeinated tea, coffee or cola with your meals as they contain tannic acid, which interferes with your absorption of iron*

<u>SUPPER</u>   complete with carbohydrates, proteins and a small amount of fat

1 glass of WATER in the early evening

<u>Late SNACK</u>   choose something that will help you sleep such as:
(only if you need it)   ½ cup plain yogurt, ½ banana, whole-wheat cereal with skim milk
or a ½ turkey sandwich.

COMPLETE YOUR DAILY BUILDING ENERGY RECORD ON PAGE 109.

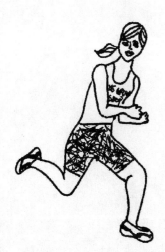

BUILDING

| **E**nergy |
| **N**utrition |
| **E**XERCISE |
| **R**est and Relaxation |
| **G**oals |
| **Y**ou |

SECTION THREE

PHYSICAL ACTIVITY

Our bodies need to move, to be Exercised.

LEARNING OBJECTIVES

After reading this Section and completing all exercises, you will

- know how to maintain your energy through physical activity
- know the best times to exercise to keep your energy up

Body Facts

Fact One
Our body likes to burn good quality fuel to be at peak energy production. We work better when we feed our body the 'good stuff'. The 'not so good stuff' slows us down and puts us in an energy slump.

Fact Two
Our body loves water. We are made up of over 60% water, so lets not forget to hydrate regularly.

Fact Three
As adults, we tend to take shallow breaths from the top of the chest instead of deep breaths from the diaphragm. Taking a few deep breaths relaxes our bodies. If we decide to smoke, we increase our risk of developing respiratory problems.

Fact Four
Our body is built to MOVE! Ever notice how tired you get when sitting all day? That's because our bodies are made up of muscles, joints, tendons, and ligaments that were designed for mobility. So start moving.

Fact Five
Not only does our body desire movement, it wants to move with ease and agility. It just feels better to be light on our feet, able to reach to the top shelf, able to open a tight lid or able to reach down and touch our toes.

Fact Six
Our bodies enjoy resistance training for a higher metabolism and more energy. Did you know that resistance training is one of the best ways to increase our metabolism as we age? It's true. Our bones love it as well.

Fact Seven
Our body likes to rest and rejuvenate. Within each 24-hour period our body likes to get 7 – 8 hours of solid sleep. This allows our body to repair, rebuild and rejuvenate.

PHYSICAL ACTIVITY FOR ENERGY

You are what you DO.

At least 21,000 Canadians die prematurely each year because they are physically inactive. That is the conclusion of a new analysis of the main diseases linked to physical inactivity, including type 2 diabetes, heart disease, stroke, colon cancer and possibly breast cancer. Researchers at York University and the University of Toronto estimated that regular physical activity would prevent about one-third of the deaths those diseases cause and would save the country more than $2.1 billion in health care costs. This information was recently published in the Nutrition Action Health Letter. We have control and can change these results.

These are just a few facts about our body that you need to keep in mind when determining your energy equation. Are we giving our bodies the right stuff to help it function like a finely tuned machine or are we neglecting our machine to eventual breakdown? Only we can decide. Pamela Smith, author of "The Energy Edge", states that:

> **"Just a ten minute walk brings an increase in energy and a decrease in tension and fatigue for as long as two hours."**

Regular physical activity helps us gear up our metabolism. This will keep our weight and our cholesterol in check. Physical activity also improves our muscle tone, boosts our immune system, helps us cope with stress and depression, relieves muscle tension, reduces our blood pressure and builds our energy reserves. So, of course, we want to build exercise into our everyday routines. We can choose from a large variety of activities that are fun and pleasurable to us. Our choices are as varied as are our tastes.

In this section we will discover what the FITT principle is, what the components of fitness and wellness are and how we can use this to increase our energy. We will also learn the benefits of physical wellness and how to add physical activity to our lives on a daily basis with JOY!

ENERGY BEGETS ENERGY!

What do I need to do to build and maintain ENERGY?

You read about the basics in Section One, but now, what do you do about it? The most important thing to know is your own body. Once you learn what your body needs and what it doesn't need, you are well on your way to building your energy. We are all very different in the amount of energy we need to take in from food and how fast our bodies metabolize food. You may have noticed how some people can eat an exorbitant amount of food and they never seem to gain a pound, while others feel that even if they just look at food, the weight will jump right on!

Metabolism refers to all the energy-requiring processes that occur in the body, such as cell growth, cell repair, and respiration. Metabolic rate is the term used to describe the speed at which the body uses energy to support these processes. The higher an individual's metabolic rate, the more food energy he or she will need to consume.

Once you understand how your body works and adapts to food and activity, you will see the results. If you are carrying excess fat, it's because your body didn't need or use it, so it stores it. This is one indicator that you are taking in too much food and not balancing that intake with a matching amount of output, i.e. "physical activity".

There are many methods of determining your ideal weight for your height, age and build. Some are very complex and must be done at a facility equipped with a hydrostatic water tank. They actually submerse you in a tank filled with water and from that they can determine the amount of body fat you have. This information will help you to see if you are average, above average or below average for the general population. Or you may undergo a fat caliper test, where skin folds are taken at various sites of your body, again to determine your "fatness". Another tool is the Body Mass Index **(BMI)** that you completed in Section Two.

Here is a basic indicator of how to determine how much you should weigh for your height. Your "ideal" body weight is 100 pounds for the first 5 feet of height, and 5 pounds per inch after that for women. For men start at 115 pounds. So for a 5 foot 6 inch woman her ideal body weight would be 130 pounds and for a 5 foot 11 inch man his ideal body weight would be 170 pounds. Now this again is just a rough indicator that doesn't take into account muscle mass or age. A very muscular person may be short in stature and heavy in muscle. Remember that muscle weighs more than fat. This is a starting point only. **You determine what is right for your body**. You will work at peak efficiency when your weight feels right for your body. Now how does energy beget energy?

The main concept to understand is **Energy Balance**.
There are two components in the energy balance equation:

Energy input (or food) = Energy output (or metabolism + physical activity)

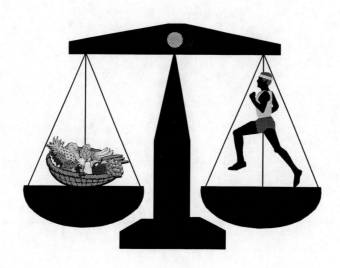

WHAT PHYSICAL ACTIVITIES HAVE YOU DONE
OVER THE PAST THREE DAYS?

Remember to include everything (walking, taking the stairs, gardening etc.)

DAY ONE:

DAY TWO:

DAY THREE:

FITT PRINCIPLE

Energy begets energy. Ever wonder why young children have so much energy? We say, "Wow, he's full of vinegar today!" or "She has energy to burn!" There are a few reasons why we as adults do not have the energy that our children and grandchildren have. The obvious reason is that children move! Very rarely will kids stand or sit still; it goes against their very nature. You hear adults constantly trying to make them sit still, but it's a losing battle. Also, as we age our metabolism does slow down. This is a completely natural process but there are ways to fight it. There is one more factor in all of this - we are programmed to slow down as we age. Ever notice at the playground, the kids are running, jumping, swinging and the adults are sitting on the benches talking. Who says we can't be playing tag, hide and

> **Remember that the fastest way to get energized is through exercise.**

seek, etc. We do concede that swinging is getting a bit tougher on the behind and there's the dizzy factor, but give it a whirl. Our society, as a whole, has been teaching us to be sedentary. We don't even get up to change the channels on the television anymore and most doors seem to open for us. We are also starting to instill this in our children by driving them to school, giving them televisions, computers and phones in their rooms. Not only will they become sedentary, you may never see them again! It's up to us to increase our energy levels by understanding how our body works and what we can do to change our energy equation for the better.

First let's discuss the FITT principle. This principle was developed to help us understand what forms of activity are beneficial to the body, how to do them and how often to do them.

F-FREQUENCY – How often should we be physically active?

It used to be that we were told to exercise at least three times a week in our maximum heart rate zone with many calculations. With the new research on physical activity things have changed for the better. We can include activity in our daily lives without joining an expensive gym or being in a fitness class wearing spandex. Studies now reveal that all forms of activity are beneficial and can be done at our own pace.

How often? The answer is simple. As often as we can!
To keep your energy at its peak - build in those physically active moments throughout your day. Take ten to twelve minutes several times a day. Get creative – some examples are:

- walk to the corner store or video store rather than taking the car
- park a few blocks from work and walk the rest of the way
- walk before and/or after lunch
- walk before and/or after that long meeting
- take the stairs instead of the elevator, etc.

> Remember, your gains in overall fitness will depend on what you put into it, so judge your results accordingly. For the best gains in overall fitness a 3 – 5 day per week commitment of sixty minutes each day will yield optimum results.

I-INTENSITY- How hard should I be exercising to get the benefit?

This also has been modified over the last number of years. Current research says that the intensity needed is dependent on your level of activity. If you have not exercised for many years, you must **start off slowly with your doctor's approval.** There are many ways to judge your intensity level; the easiest and most common is the talk test. While you are walking, mowing, gardening, climbing stairs, jogging or swimming, you should be able to sustain a conversation without gasping for air. You should feel like you are getting a benefit. Your body will tell you if you are working too hard or not hard enough. Our muscles adapt very quickly, so it is important to keep varying the intensity to reap the benefits.

We have learned that exercise at a **moderate intensity** gives a better overall health benefit. We seem to get all the positives for our bodies and certainly **for our energy** with none of the possible damage to our joints and muscles that high impact activities can sometimes bring. So look for the low-impact aerobics, brisk walking, swimming, cross country skiing, cycling, etc. and get all the possible benefits.

Take a look at the following study that shows that all things in moderation is still the best advice.

From the Journal of American Medical Association
(Age adjusted death rates per 10,000 people)

Death Rates by Fitness Groups, Women

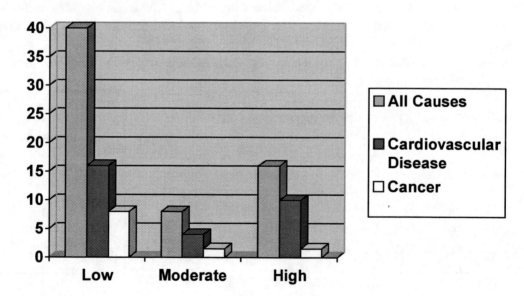

Death Rates by Fitness Groups, Men

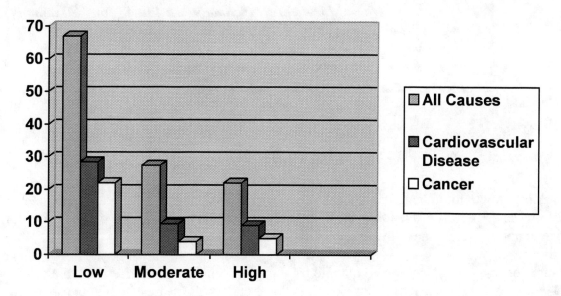

T-TIME- **How long do I need to be active?**

Things have changed in the world of lifestyle choices. We used to preach that people exercise a minimum of 20 minutes consecutively in their target heart rate zone to achieve benefits. It is true that you will achieve cardiovascular benefits by doing this, but there are alternatives.

The new research indicates that it is the **cumulative activity that you do each day that adds up** as well. So, if you walk to the store for ten minutes, walk up 5 flights of stairs, mow your grass and do some light gardening you've got your 20-30 minutes of beneficial activity for that day. Don't despair! Keep adding up the time of your physical activity and you may surprise yourself at the end of the day.

"Low Fat Living" by Robert K. Cooper and Leslie L. Cooper, say it best when they propose their 'Four Fives and a Ten Plan'. This is doable even for we "busy" folks. It goes like this
- 5 minutes of easy physical activity in the morning – either before or after your balanced breakfast
- 5 to 10 minutes walk before lunch
- 5 to 10 minutes walk after lunch
- 5 minutes of easy stretching or muscle toning when you get home
- 10 – 20 minutes walk after supper

> **Using more oxygen to do moderate exercise within a half hour of eating means that our food will "burn hotter" using more calories.**
> **This means fewer calories are left over to be stored as fat.**

> *Research at Harvard Medical School's Institute for Circadian Physiology has shown that every time you use muscular activity, you increase your energy and alertness. So by just taking a few minutes here and there – you are still getting a solid metabolic boost.*

T-TYPE – What kind of activity should I do?

Any kind of activity is beneficial. The main message is to move! Sitting at a computer all day does not lend itself to movement. Think of our ancestors who had to go out and hunt for their dinner, chop firewood, make the fire, cook the food and then clean up.

We are not suggesting that you go out and try to shoot a chicken for dinner, but think about what you could do to be more active. For example, don't park in the nearest spot at the shopping mall, chose one far away and carry your groceries to it. Just the act of carrying and lifting groceries will get your heart rate going. The main idea is to be more active generally and then try something new. Find things that you enjoy and don't be afraid to keep trying. Once you feel your fitness level improving it opens up many choices of other activities. Try ballroom dancing, join an aerobics class, take up kick boxing**…the sky is the limit!**

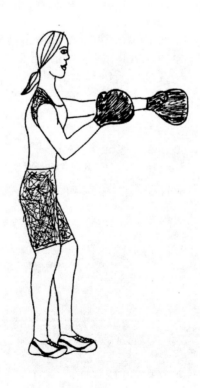

FIVE COMPONENTS OF PHYSICAL FITNESS

"If exercise could be packaged into a pill,
it would be the single most prescribed and beneficial medicine in the nation."
Robert Butler. M.D.

The research in the area of physical activity is indisputable. It is essential to keeping your body healthy and fine tuned. We are going to focus on how to use physical activity to gain more energy for your life. In order to do this we need to understand the basics of physical fitness and how it relates to our bodies. There are five main components of fitness. We will discuss each of them and give examples of how they can fit into your lifestyle.

1. Aerobic Fitness

Aerobic fitness is basically how efficient your heart and lungs are at getting the oxygen we breathe to the working muscles. This system, the cardiovascular system, is extremely important to our heart health. There are many benefits to using and developing this system for energy. **The more efficient the system, the more energy we will have.** The reason for this is that if our aerobic system is at peak efficiency our resting heart rate will be lower, our blood pressure will decrease, our recovery time will be lowered and our ability to transport oxygenated blood to our working muscles will increase. All of these factors lead to more energy production at a faster, easier rate! In order to develop our aerobic fitness, we need to move our large muscle groups, the legs for example, for a period of time to achieve an increase in aerobic capacity.

Your choices of aerobic activities are wide and varied. We encourage you to choose a variety of things you like to do, things that you can and will fit into your busy daily schedule. Remember you can spread your aerobic activities throughout your day. We've listed some ideas for you – but get creative – do what you love and will continue to commit yourself to doing.

Let's take a look at <u>some</u> of the wonderful aerobic exercise choices we have:

Walking
Something we can all do at any age and any fitness level. Our injury risk is very low. Start off slowly and increase your pace, as you feel comfortable. If you walk at a slow to moderate pace, increase your time to get the best benefits. Remember to dress comfortably and wear a good walking runner.

> *"My advice is to walk whenever you can. It's free, costs nothing.*
> *It not only makes you live longer and feel better,*
> *it also keeps you looking trim."*
> George Burns –" How to Live to be 100 – or More"

One way to increase the number of STEPS you take each day is described on the following page.

WALK YOUR WAY TO GREATER ENERGY

It's easy, it's cheap, and we can do it anywhere. The benefits are life long and have been proven beyond a doubt. So what's stopping us? Let's get more STEPS into each and every day. Add them in anywhere and everywhere. Many people have *GAINED ENERGY*, lost weight, lost inches, and are in overall better health by adding extra STEPS to their day.

Walking is great at any fitness level. It's an **excellent energy builder** as it helps us build stamina and strength. So, even if you feel you are 'out of shape', walking is for you! Start out slowly walking at your own pace just a block or two. Remember that even ten to fifteen minutes will help you feel and look better and, best of all, will increase your **energy**. Gradually speed up your pace and lengthen your time. To warm your muscles as you begin your walk, simply walk at a slower pace for the first block or so, then stop and run through the stretching exercises – briefly. Remember to hold your stretches – do not bounce. When you've finished your walk, take the time to slowly stretch your leg muscles, you can hold the stretches longer as your muscles are warm. If walking is your main exercise try to walk more often and for longer periods or time. As you become more fit and want more challenge, pick up the pace, add an incline, or find some stairs.

Ensure you are wearing good footwear with proper arch support. Caring for our feet is an investment in our future quality of life. We want to protect our muscles and joints from damage. If you have knee problems try to stay on the grass versus walking on concrete.

Walking, for many of us, is more fun with a partner. When Wendy and Bev are out walking, their mouths get as much exercise as their bodies. If you don't have a partner, we recommend you count your steps using a PEDOMETER. Pedometers, get the step counting kind, are inexpensive and can be purchased at most fitness equipment stores. With a Pedometer you can compete with yourself. You could set a goal, add more steps each week, and even wear your pedometer all day.

Another idea Bev has used is to buy a 'walking tape' and listen to the directions and walk to the beat.

TIPS
- *MAKE IT FUN!*
- *keep a journal -- make a note on Your Daily Energy Building Record (found at the end of this book)*
- *socialize – find a partner whenever possible*
- *look for opportunities everywhere – get creative*

Treadmill

If you can't walk outside, walk inside. Learn how to use the equipment safely. We know walking is good for everyone – all ages and all levels of fitness. Wear your pedometer. Start off slowly; build up your length of time, your speed, and your rate of incline as you build your stamina and your fitness level.

Jogging or Running

This does give us a good workout, but we do add an element of risk. Be sure you are in good shape before you decide to run or jog. Ensure you have excellent footwear and, to help prevent joint injury, do your running on surfaces that have some give to them like a proper running track, grass or dirt.

Stair Climbing or Bench Stepping

Excellent choices. Stairs are certainly easy to find. Start off with ten minutes, then slowly increase your time as your stamina and strength increases. Good for all ages and levels of fitness.

Cycling or Stationary Cycling

A wonderful way to increase your energy is to cycle the great outdoors. Good for the whole family. This one also has less stress on our joints. On days when you can't get out, try the stationary bicycle. Learn how to operate the equipment safely, log your time and your speed. Increase the level of difficulty as you build your strength. This equipment is good for all adults, including older people, people with joint problems, those who are overweight, during pregnancy, and for those just beginning to exercise.

Swimming or Aquasizes

Do this at your own pace. Join a daily, biweekly or weekly class. You can push hard or go easy. Listen to your body and decide. This is especially good for people with arthritis or other joint problems as there is no weight on the joints. Swimming or Aquasizes are also good during pregnancy, for people recovering from injury, and for older people.

Cross Country Skiing

This gives us a full body workout. If you've got snow, you're good to go. But, we can do this inside or outside, even simulate the movements in the pool. We can choose our own speed and our own level of difficulty.

Rowing

Rowing helps us build overall body strength and aerobic fitness. Again start off slowly and work your way up to working harder for longer periods.

Jumping Rope

This one gets our heart rate up fairly fast. When you have worked up to a good level of fitness you can work this one in as an added section of your exercise fun.

Mini-Trampoline

A Mini Trampoline doesn't take up too much room. You can take it indoors or out. Be sure that you have enough space and can do this safely. Go at your own pace.

Aerobics

Very popular and an excellent choice. We highly recommend you only do low-impact aerobics to ensure you are protecting your joints. Good for all ages and fitness levels. Remember to go at your own pace. You should always be able to carry on a conversation. If you can't talk - slow down!

2. Flexibility

Flexibility is defined as the ability of a joint to move through its full range of motion. As we age we may lose some flexibility, but you'll be happy to know that this component of fitness is the easiest and fastest to regain. Just a few mild stretches each day will increase your level of flexibility. With more flexibility you will have smoother and more efficient flow of movement. What this leads to, of course, is conserving energy that you can use elsewhere. Include stretching regularly, before and after any physical activity. Try a yoga class.

3. Muscular Endurance

Muscular endurance refers to the number of times a muscle or group of muscles can repeatedly exert a force without fatiguing, or the ability to sustain a given level of muscle tension. An example of muscular endurance would be carrying a large suitcase over a distance. Our muscular endurance helps us with our posture and with injury prevention. With proper muscular endurance, we will be able to do activities for a longer period of time before we become fatigued. Increasing our endurance means increasing our energy! Muscular endurance activities include light resistance training, calisthenics, cycling, pilates, swimming, hiking, and walking.

4. Muscular Strength

By definition muscular strength is the maximum amount of tension/force that a muscle or a muscle group can exert in a single contraction. This doesn't mean that we expect you to run out to the gym and try to bench-press 500 pounds. What it does mean is that for energy purposes muscular strength is important.

Strong and balanced muscle groups help us immensely with day-to-day activities. Strong muscles help us conserve energy. The ability to pick up a heavy suitcase or open a tight fitting lid are examples of muscular strength. Muscle tissue burns more calories than fat, so the higher the muscle content the better energy user we are. As we age we lose muscle content naturally. About 30 percent of our total number of muscle cells disappear between ages 20 – 70.

Through strength training, we can increase our metabolism by as much as 15 –20 percent. So, let's get active with weight bearing activities and build our energy! Some examples of strength building activities are weight training, power lifting, Pilates, calisthenics, use of tubing or bands, and general lifting.

5. Body Composition

We refer to body composition as the fifth component of fitness as it is an indicator of overall health and wellness. Body composition refers to the amount of water, fat and lean body tissue (muscle and bone) that our bodies have. We are aiming for a high proportion of lean body tissue and a low proportion of fat. This healthy composition will maintain our health and lower our risk of diseases that are associated with obesity.

BENEFITS OF PHYSICAL ACTIVITY

> *We need to be physically active every day if we are to achieve and maintain physical fitness and good health. Regular physical activity is essential for healthy and vigorous living. To a large extent WE ARE WHAT WE DO-- weak or strong, energetic or lethargic.*

It is clear that being physically active has many benefits as it:

- *gives us more **energy boosting oxygen***
- *boosts the flow of oxygenated blood to our brain (**think more clearly, creatively**)*
- *releases those beta-endorphins – promoting a sense of **well being***
- *reduces the incidence of heart disease and hypertension*
- *increases the production of the 'good' cholesterol HDL*
- *improves our ability to **sleep soundly***
- *gives us a more positive **attitude***
- *improved work **performance***
- *promotes less strain and tension*
- *provides **greater stamina**, strength, endurance, and coordination*
- *increases joint flexibility*
- ***reduces chronic fatigue***
- *results in an improved and more efficient circulatory system*

We have discussed the FITT principle, basic components of fitness, ways to include activity into our daily lives, and the basics of how our body uses food for energy production.

Now the question is: What are you going to do with this knowledge?

WATCH WATER WALK WEIGHTS WONDERFUL

WALK
--as often as you can!

I love to exercise and move my body.
I have stamina, strength, endurance and coordination.
I have energy to spare.

My notes on Physical Activity:

I am going to build Physical Activity into every day by:

Building Energy Through Muscle Toning

MYTHS *of Muscle Toning*

Before we get into all of the benefits of muscle toning for energy production, let's discuss some of the common myths about resistance training.

MYTH *"Weight training makes you muscle bound."*

You may notice that some people who are involved with heavy weight training for competition seem very muscle bound and inflexible. This can occur if you are not warming up properly, stretching the muscle groups in between sets of exercises and if you are not doing the exercise properly. Each exercise that you do should go through the full range of motion that the joint is capable of. This will actually increase the flexibility of that joint.

MYTH *"Muscle turns to fat if you stop training."*

The first thing to understand is that muscle and fat are two different types of tissues in the body. One cannot "turn" into the other. When you are participating in resistance training to build muscle (hypertrophy), the muscle cells will increase in size. When you stop exercising your muscles the muscle cells atrophy or decrease in size. This also occurs if you are bed ridden for a long period of time. Now, you may notice that some people gain fat after they stop doing resistance training. This is largely due to the fact that they continue to keep eating the same number of calories as when they were training and therefore are storing more calories in the form of fat.

MYTH *"Weight training is a great way to trim fat off specific body parts."*

First, let's clear something up. Spot reduction is physiologically impossible, yet this myth is one of the most popular and still believed by many people. You could do 1,000 sit ups per day and still have fat stores in your abdominal region. You may not like it, but it's the truth. Fat is not used from the deposits near the exercising muscle, but from the fatty acids carried in the blood and the fat droplets stored within the muscle.

TRUTHS of Muscle Toning

Listed below are some great truths about the benefit of strength training and specifically to metabolism and energy production.

- Lowers our resting blood pressure.

- Increases our high-density lipoproteins (HDL) - the type that helps prevent coronary heart disease as blood lipids (fats) are favorably altered.

- Improves our sense of well-being and self-esteem.

- Reduces the strain of daily activities and chores.

- Prevents injuries in physical activities.

- Muscle mass is increased and body fat is slightly dissipated.

- Look smaller and trimmer at the same weight as muscle is denser than fat.

- Resting metabolic rate is raised as our extra muscle tissue may consume more calories at rest than fat does.

- Gain muscular strength in the large muscle groups in our legs, arms, stomach, and back helping us in our everyday activities such as walking, lifting, and sitting.

- Tight, toned muscles don't sag.

- Muscular strength, endurance, and efficiency are increased.

Now, specifically, what is the benefit of muscle toning through resistance training with regards to **energy production**? In Section One, 'How Our Body Works and How Our Body is Fueled', we discussed the energy stored and available in the muscle cell itself. At the cellular level, increased stores of ATP and CP occur as a direct result of strength training. Not only is there extra energy available to the muscle during exercise, but also the release of energy occurs more readily due to increased efficiency in the system to break down ATP. This helps us in our daily lives on many levels and will lead to a general increase in energy available to us. In our Energy Equation, **resistance training is a big plus for our increase in energy reserves.**

So, what kinds of resistance-training activities should I do and how do I get started? The first thing that you should know is that you don't have to run out and buy an expensive gym membership. You can use virtually anything as your resistance. Your own body weight, even soup cans, is an excellent start.

RESISTANCE TRAINING GUIDELINES

Note: It is recommended that you take a
24 to 48 hour rest period between training sessions.
The length of time of the rest period depends on the type and intensity of the training.
The harder you work, the more rest required between training sessions.

- **Start slowly with little or no resistance.**

- **Sometimes just your own body weight is enough resistance to begin a program.**

- **Start with your large muscle groups and then move to your smaller muscle groups.**

- **Maintain a 'neutral spine' position throughout each movement.**

- **Keep your actions slow and controlled and breathe. We need to oxygenate our muscles to work. Inhale on the relaxation phase of the movement and exhale on the exertion (contraction) phase.**

- **Use the full range of motion; this will alleviate the fear of becoming 'muscle bound'.**

- **Stretch the muscle group that you have exercised at the end of that muscle group activity.**

- **Drink water before, during and following all exercise.**

- **Start off the activity with a warm up.**

- **Seek the advice of a professional personal trainer when beginning a program.**

We have included some basic movements in this workbook to get you started on a resistance-training program. Remember to start with learning the movements first. Our muscles need to learn and adapt to the activities we ask them to perform. **Proper technique in resistance training is key for optimal benefit and to decrease the risk of injury.** You will experience some discomfort when you first begin a resistance training activity. Do not despair. This is a normal sensation due to the process of muscle re-building and it will dissipate over time.

WARM UPS – COOL DOWNS – FLEXIBILITY
AND STRETCHING

One of the biggest complaints we hear from people is that exercise hurts. **Well, it doesn't have to and in fact, it shouldn't**. The days of "feel the burn" are gone, thank goodness. If the physical activity you have chosen is hurting you, you are either doing something wrong or working too hard or too fast. Stop and seek help before you injure yourself and then become unable to exercise. If you haven't included activity in your daily life for quite some time it is strongly recommended that you **seek the approval of your physician first**. Get a full physical examination and then discuss your activity choices with your doctor before you begin.

There are a few things that you can do to decrease the chance of injury during your physical activity. The first is a proper warm up. Our muscles need to be warmed up before we do any type of activity. This includes 5 – 10 minutes of light movement followed by both active and passive stretching.

Warm ups

To begin any activity you should first **warm up** the muscles and joints with light aerobic activity. Many of our joints are synovial joints. For example, the shoulders, elbows and knees all have fluid inside of them that aids in mobility. We need to warm these joints up in order to release the synovial fluid to protect us from injury. We also need to move our large muscle groups in our legs to increase our heart rate and therefore pump more blood to our working muscles. For example, you can do a light walk, march on the spot, ride a bike or walk up some stairs. Anything to get you moving. Remember to start slow and work your way up. The entire warm up could only be 5 – 10 minutes focusing on light movement. Once you have warmed the muscles, do some light stretches. Focus on the muscle groups that you will be using during your chosen activity with short held stretches totaling 2-3 minutes of your warm-up time. Static stretches are slow, controlled, held stretches. Don't bounce! Hold each stretch for about 5-10 seconds, breathe naturally, and remember this is just the warm up. This form of stretching can be interspersed with active stretches as well.

Cool downs

In the **cool down** phase of activity you can do a variety of stretches. Hold them for a longer period of time, as your muscles will be very warm following activity. Keep the stretches static in nature. Hold with no bouncing and hold the stretch for 30-90 seconds each. This is where the most gains in **flexibility** will be achieved.

The following are some suggested stretches for most types of activity:

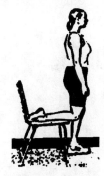
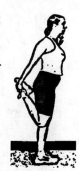

Quadriceps (front of the thigh) Standing Stretch- It is very important to stretch the front of the thigh before any activity. These muscles need to be stretched, as they are used daily in walking, climbing, and all frontal plane movement. Using a wall or chair for support, stand tall, bend your knee and if you can reach, hold your ankle. If you can't reach your ankle use the chair behind you to rest your knee on. For a further stretch in this position push forward through your hip. This will give you a full stretch of all of those front muscles. Do not bounce! Hold for about ten seconds. Breathe normally. Repeat on the other leg.

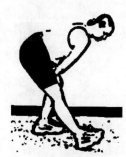

Hamstring (back of thigh) Standing Stretch- Start in a standing position. Place one leg out in front. Lean forward toward the extended leg. Rest your hands on the other leg, which should be bent. Hold, release and repeat on the other side. Remember not to hold your breath.

Standing Calf Stretch- These are very strong muscles and can get stiff and sore, so use this stretch. Stand with arms outstretched. Lean against a wall. Reach one leg back and bend the front knee. Bend your elbows and lean further into the wall. When you feel the muscle stretching – hold. Do this with a straight extended leg, and then a slightly bent extended leg. Try to keep your heel pressed to the floor. Repeat for both legs.

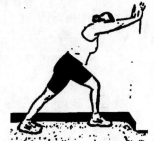

Shoulder Stretch- There are many ways to warm up and stretch the shoulder joint. First stand tall and clasp your hands together, then stretch your arms overhead. Hold. Take your hands behind your back. Clasp your hands together and stretch - opening up your chest area. Hold. Now clasp your hands out in front, stretch your arms out and think of spreading your shoulder blades. Hold. These stretches actually stretch many muscle groups in your upper body.

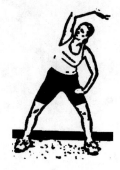

Side Bend Stretch- This stretch will warm up your large muscle groups in the upper and lower back region. Standing with your feet slightly wider than shoulder width apart and with your knees slightly bent, reach over to one side. You can place your hand on your knee for support of your spine. Hold. Release and then repeat on the other side.

MUSCLE TONING ACTIVITIES

Remember to do your WARM-UP and COOL-DOWN stretches.

Building ENDURANCE

Lighter weights and higher repetitions are recommended to build your endurance. Your goal here is to tone and not to build muscle. **Start with one set of 15 to 25 repetitions.** Once that becomes easy you can add a second set and even a third over time if you wish.

Building MUSCLE and increasing MUSCLE STRENGTH

If your goal is to build and strengthen your muscles, use heavier resistance and fewer repetitions. **Start with one set of 8 to 12 repetitions.** When your muscles have adapted, increase the number of sets to two or three.

We recommend that you do some easy stretching of the muscles that you have worked each time you complete all the exercises for that muscle group. Then, after the entire workout session, end with full deep stretching. Enjoy!

> **Remember: You must give your muscles a rest between workouts to allow them time to rebuild. Take a 24-48 hour rest period between resistance training sessions. The amount of time of rest depends on the type and intensity of the training. The harder you work your muscles, the longer your rest period needs to be.**

Lower Body:

Squats- This form of activity is very basic and easy to perform. When you execute the squat properly you will be working many different muscle groups of the thighs and buttocks. You can perform it with a barbell or by holding dumbbells or soup cans in your hands. Stand with your feet slightly wider than shoulder width apart and your toes

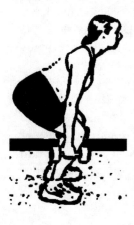

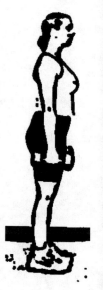

turned out slightly. It is a good idea to place a chair behind you so that when you squat down your buttocks will slightly touch the chair. This will do two things. You will not bend down too low; possibly injuring your knees and the chair will be a support if you need to rest. Now, allow your knees and hips to flex until your thighs are parallel to the floor. Keep your back straight throughout the lowering phase by jutting out your behind as required. Then squeeze and push yourself up to the standing position. Breathing properly is always important. Breathe in on the downward phase of the movement and breathe out on exertion when pushing back up to the standing position. If you have knee problems don't go down as far.

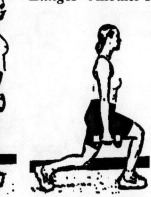

Lunges- Another staple muscle toning activity is the lunge. When done properly it will shape the muscles of your buttocks, thighs, and calves. Start in a standing position feet slightly apart and facing straight forward. You can use no resistance, a barbell, dumbbells, or soup cans. You decide. Then lunge forward with a large step with one leg and bend the knee to a parallel position with the other leg relaxed and almost touching the floor. Then push the front leg back to the full standing position. Initiate this movement from the heel of the foot, not the toe. Repeat on the other leg and continue alternating legs. If you are experiencing any knee pain, stop and try again but don't bend your knees as far. Keep it simple and pain free.

Calf raises- The lower leg is also very valuable to tone. We use it every time we point our toes. The best way to build strength in this muscle is to raise yourself up onto your toes. So, starting in a standing position, with resistance or not, press up until you are on your toes, release and repeat. If you have trouble balancing, hold on to a chair or to the wall for support. You can add resistance by holding dumbbells or soup cans.

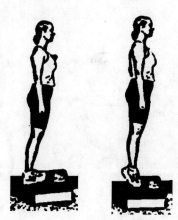

Upper Body

Chest (Pectoral) Muscles- There are numerous ways to exercise the pectoral muscle group. We will discuss the bench press. You can lie on your back on an exercise bench, a hard bed, or the floor to do this activity. Again you can use no resistance, dumbbells, barbell, or soup cans. If your back is arching you can bend your knees. This will help keep your back flat. Start with elbows bent and by your side and extend your arms up, concentrating on

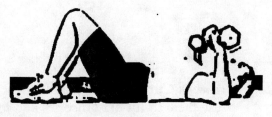

squeezing the chest muscles on the way up. Breathe out as you are pushing up and breathe in as you come back down, bending the elbows. If you are uncomfortable with this exercise, you can try push-ups for similar results.

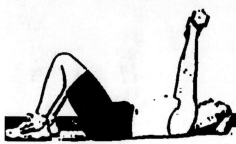

Back (Upper and Lower)- There are many ways to facilitate back strength. The one-arm bent over row exercise is effective and fairly easy to execute. Start by resting

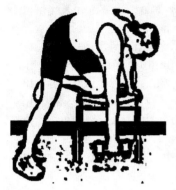

your knee and arm on a bench, the edge of a bed, or a chair. With the resistance in your other arm, initiate the lift from your lower back, pulling your elbow up towards the ceiling. Once your elbow is slightly above the parallel level hold and squeeze. Slowly let your arm drop down to full extension. Your breathing is important. Breathe in on the lowering phase and breathe out on the upward lift. Do your set(s) and then repeat for the other side.

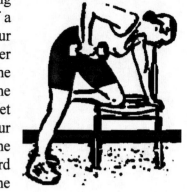

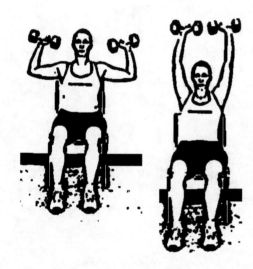

Shoulders- The "military press" can be completed either standing or sitting. Start with the resistance at shoulder level. Press straight up. Hold and release. Breathe out going up and breathe in coming down.

Biceps Curls- Biceps are the muscles at the front of the upper arm. We use them to lift our groceries and to do any forward elbow flexion. Do a simple biceps curl from a standing position. Start with feet shoulder width apart and maintain a neutral spine throughout the movement (do not bend forward or backward during the lift). Extend your arms down by your sides, holding the resistance. Breathe out as you initiate the move from the bicep and continue pulling all the way up to full flexion. Breathe in as you release slowly down to the starting position.

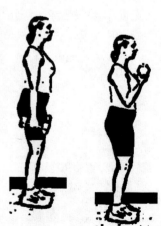

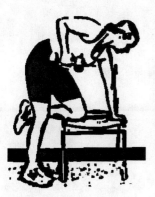

Tricep Kickbacks- The triceps are located at the back of the upper arm. It is fairly underused, as we don't walk swinging our arms backwards. We do however want to exercise this muscle to balance our well-used biceps muscles. Start in the same position that you did with the one-arm bent over row. This time raise the elbow up to parallel and hold it there. Just extend your elbow, hold, squeeze, and release back down. Breathe out on the extension and in when returning to the start position. Complete your set(s), then repeat for the other arm.

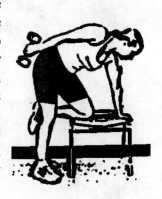

Wrist Curls- In our computer age it is more important than ever to strengthen the many small flexors and extensors in our lower arm. To do this, hold the resistance in your hands and be in a seated position. Rest your forearms on your knees and hang your wrists over the end of your knees. Curl the wrists both ways. Start with your palms facing the ceiling. Use your muscles to curl your knuckles toward your forearm. Do your set(s), then reverse, placing your palms down to the floor and curl up.

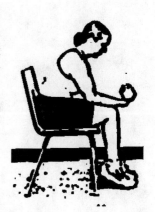

Breathing is so important during our exercise as our <u>muscles need oxygen</u>. Breathe in with muscle relaxation and breathe out with muscle exertion.

WATCH WATER WALK WEIGHTS WONDERFUL

WEIGHTS

--build strength and muscular endurance!

I feel strong.
My body can easily get me where I want to go.
I have energy for the whole day and into the evening.

My notes on using Weights:

I will build more Muscle Toning exercises into my weekly routine by:

BUILDING ENERGY THROUGH EXERCISE

It boils down to smart choices, over and over again.
The healthier you can maintain your body through smart food choices, along with supplements,
exercise, and restful sleep - the more ENERGIZED YOU WILL BE.

In our research we have found that when we build exercise throughout our day, we maintain our energy levels and keep our metabolism burning.

An energy begets energy day could look like this:

Morning
Park or get off the bus early and get a **10-minute walk** to work.
At morning break do a **series of stretches and deep breathing** before your energy snack.
At lunch break **walk up and down the stairs for 10 minutes** before your energy lunch.
After you eat take a **10-minute walk** outside.

Afternoon
At afternoon break do a **series of strength and muscular endurance** activities in your office or in the bathroom, with or without resistance.
After work get off the bus a few stops early and **walk** the rest of the way.
While making or helping with supper do some **standing calisthenics**.

Evening
Play a game with your children, go to the park, do some yard work or housework.
If you choose to watch TV, do **exercises or household chores** during commercials.
Go for a **walk** after supper.
Before you go to bed enjoy a **20-minute beginners yoga** tape or a **meditation** tape.
If possible have an intimate 10 – 15 minutes or more with your partner.

Get a good night's sleep.

*Find YOUR DAILY BUILDING ENERGY RECORD at the end of this book. Duplicate and use this sheet every day until **building energy** becomes a daily habit.*

Today – How many minutes of aerobic activity did you get? _____

Did you do any strength and muscular endurance activities? _____

Did you increase flexibility? _____

Remember – take one day at a time. Today -- if you missed out don't worry about it,
just take the next day – one day at a time and enjoy your energy.

MY NOTES:

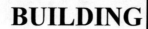

BUILDING | **E**nergy
Nutrition
Exercise
REST
Goals
You

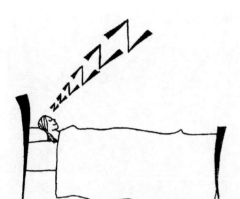

SECTION FOUR

REJUVENATION THROUGH REST

Our body and our mind need sleep and rest to repair and rebuild.

LEARNING OBJECTIVE

After you have read this Section and completed the exercises, you will

- **understand your body's need for sleep and know how to re-energize yourself through sleep, rest, relaxation, and fun**

REJUVENATION THROUGH <u>REST</u>

Peaceful sleep is essential for health and well being because during sleep, the body's restorative functions take place.

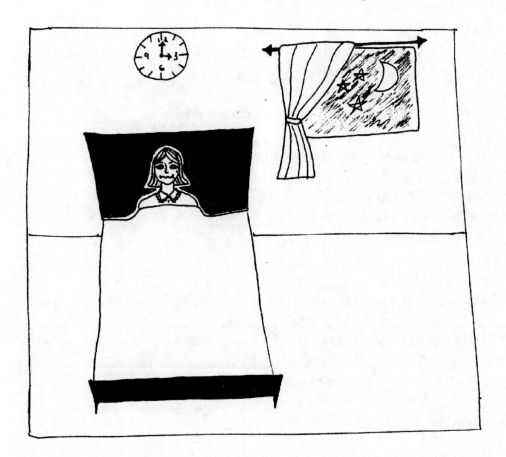

DID YOU KNOW THAT….

- one out of every four people report significant sleep problems
- many industrial accidents and over 500,000 car accidents a year in North America may be caused by sleepiness
- people with chronic poor sleep are 2.5 times more likely to suffer a car accident
- up to 20% of those who work shifts suffer from insomnia due to upsetting their 'biological clock'
- daytime performance can be adversely affected by lack of sleep
- the older people get, the more likely they are to suffer from sleeping problems
- although 8 hours is considered a 'normal' amount of sleep, some people need as few as 6 or as many as 10

SLEEP PATTERNS - SELF ASSESSMENT

Complete the following assessment.

1. What time do you usually go to bed on weeknights? _____
2. What time do you usually go to bed on weekend nights? _____
3. Do you fall asleep immediately? _____
   after 20 minute? _____
   after 40 minutes? _____
4. Do you get up at close to the same time each weekday? _____
   each weekend? _____
5. Is your bed big enough for you to roll over in, to be comfortable in?
   _____
6. Is your bedroom dark? _____
7. Is your bedroom cool enough? _____
8. Do you read in bed? _____
9. Do you watch T.V. in bed? _____
10. Do you work in bed? _____
11. What do you eat during the evenings and especially before you go to bed?
    _____
12. What do you drink during the evenings and especially before you go to bed?
    _____
13. Do you drink any caffeine beverage after 6:00 p.m.? _____
    what? and how much? _____
14. Do you wake up during the night? _____
    about when? _____
15. Do you wake up during the night worrying about work? _____
16. How many times a night do you wake up? _____
17. Can you get right back to sleep after waking? _____
18. Do you exercise in the evening? _____
19. What time in the evening do you exercise? _____
    for how long? _____
    at what intensity? _____
20. How soon after exercise do you go to bed? _____
21. How do you "prepare" yourself for bed? _____
    _____
    _____
    _____

REJUVENATION THROUGH REST

We have heard a lot about the benefits of proper nutrition, drinking enough water and getting enough physical activity. Now we want to look at how much sleep affects our quality of life and specifically our energy levels. Did you know that sleep deprivation is becoming an epidemic in our society today? Our body needs sleep to repair and rebuild itself. We spend nearly one third of our life sleeping and that adds up to about 25 years! Sleep is not merely "time out" from daily life. It's an active state essential for mental and physical restoration. Within a 24-hour daily cycle our bodies require about 8 hours of sleep. Because each person is different, some require more sleep, some less, each day. **For the majority of us 8 hours is what we need.**

All of us go through sleep patterns throughout our sleep cycle. Research tells us that there are two distinct phases in the sleep cycle, ***non- REM*** and ***REM sleep*** (REM rapid eye movement). Even if we don't remember, everyone dreams while sleeping.

There are four stages in **non-REM sleep** that we go through during our sleep pattern:

Stage 1
When we are first falling asleep we may jerk and wake ourselves and/or our partners up. This is called the "hypnagogic startle". These jerks are normal and the frequency varies among people, but there is no cause for alarm.
Stage 2
Once we slip into Stage 2 we can still be easily woken.
Stage 3
Once we are in Stage 3 we are in a deeper state of sleep.
Stage 4
When our body arrives at Stage 4 our heart rate and breathing becomes very stable. It is very difficult to be brought to a state of full wakefulness without a powerful stimulus. We would, however, be able to be brought to full wakefulness by an alarm of some sort, whether it's a baby's cry or a smoke detector.

Interspersed with non-REM sleep is REM sleep. REM sleep accounts for about 20 percent of the sleep cycle. REM sleep is very different. Internally our bodies are active, with increased brainwaves, heart rate, and a faster breathing rate. Externally our limbs are in a deep, almost paralyzing state of relaxation. As noted in the name, REM sleep is identified by the rapid eye movement noticeably visible under the eyelids. We go through these stages every time we sleep.

Each one of us has our own internal clock, commonly called our *biorhythm*. Most of us operate on a schedule of a wakeful period during daylight hours and a sleep period during the evening. This is because of our hormonal makeup. People that work shift work have great difficulty in adjusting their own internal clock to change to a schedule that doesn't fit this natural rhythm. We also experience different biorhythms throughout the day when we have highs and lows. These changes occur naturally with the changes in our body temperature. Temperature begins to rise before waking and continues to do so as the day progresses, reaching a peak in the afternoon before it starts to decline. It reaches its lowest ebb in the early hours of the morning, which is the time of day when most deaths occur. Physical skill and intellectual performance rise and fall in line with body temperature changes.

We now know the basics of sleep patterns and why our bodies require the proper amount of sleep for us to function at peak efficiency. We also know that our body has natural highs and lows throughout the day and these facts will all help us in building our energy.

HOW DO WE GET A GOOD NIGHT'S SLEEP?

Many of us fight going to bed at a time when our body requires sleep. With the invention of electricity, night can stay light and trick our body into a wakeful state. In the old days when it got dark, it got really dark and we went to bed. Another invention that keeps us from sleep is, of course, the television. We watch endless episodes of our favorite shows. Or even worse, we end our day with a newscast that disturbs us greatly, instead of allowing our bodies to wind down for sleep! As children, staying up late was a reward for good behavior. We thought that staying up late was a rite of passage into adulthood. Now as adults all our body wants is to go to bed early.

The first step in getting enough sleep, to re-build the energy we lost during the day, is to listen to our body. When you exhibit the signs of tiredness (yawning, eyes shutting, the need to lie down) try going to bed - even if that starts to happen at 9:00 p.m.! Remember what we discussed in the section on physical activity and how energy begets energy? We also looked at how children have energy to burn due to their high activity level throughout the day. Well here is another piece to the puzzle answered - when do children go to bed? How many hours of sleep do they get? We are not saying that you have to go back in time and become a child again, but we are saying that we can learn about our own energy reserves by looking at those who have energy.

There are many books available that discuss numerous ways to increase our quality of sleep to help us in our daily lives. They all seem to have some common threads that we will look at now and discuss.

Be Clock Driven

The experts all agree that going to bed and rising at approximately the same time everyday, including weekends will greatly enhance our quality of sleep. The time that we go to bed is very important in this equation. Try going to bed an hour earlier for one week and see how your body reacts to the extra sleep. Continuing this practice will train our internal clock and enable us to be at our peak energy levels throughout the day.

Develop Sleep Hygiene

Sleep Sanctuary
The other common recommendations involve training ourselves to follow regular patterns that will help us prepare for sleep. Things like the size and type of bed we sleep in to what we eat and drink prior to sleep are all factors. Our bedroom should be our **'sleep sanctuary'**! It is best not to have a television in this room. The television could cause us to stay up later than our body wants. Let's use our bedroom for sex and sleep only, not as a multi purpose room.

Suggestions for setting up our bedroom for sleep are to:
- set the temperature at around **19 degrees** Celsius, (that's about **68 degrees** Fahrenheit)
- keep the room **dark** (heavier window coverings)
- keep the bedroom a **quiet** place to sleep
- ensure that the **bed is large enough** to roll around in without hitting your sleep partner
- ensure that the **bed is just right** for you - not too soft, not too hard, not too small. It pays to invest in a good mattress with a separate spring system if possible for different body weights.

What to Eat and Drink before Bed

Now, with regards to eating and drinking prior to sleep it is agreed that caffeine consumption should be stopped by midday. That means **no caffeine** in any food products, coffee, teas, chocolate, cola-type sodas, cocoa, and any hidden caffeine in anything. Did you know that North Americans consume 400 million cups of coffee each day? We must choose our food and drinks very carefully before we go to bed.

It has been proven that eating high fat and high sugar foods prior to sleep, disturb our sleep pattern in a negative way. So much for the chips and candy before bed! On the opposite side of the coin going to bed hungry will disturb your sleep pattern as well. So, what are we supposed to do? According to Pamela Smith, author of "The Energy Edge" -- a great bedtime snack is a small bowl of whole grain cereal with low fat milk or half a turkey sandwich, a piece of cheese or a banana with skim milk. Please refer to ENERGIZING SNACKS on page 39.

Nicotine and Alcohol

Nicotine and/or alcohol consumption prior to sleep are also proven troublemakers. Nicotine is a stimulant and smokers can take longer to fall asleep. While alcohol may seem like a nice way to end the evening, it will contribute to a more fragile sleep.

Strenuous Exercise

It has also been proven that strenuous exercise too close to bedtime will adversely affect our sleep patterns. Exercise in the evening should finish at least two full hours before bedtime.

Pre Sleep Rituals

Train your body to sleep. Send it the right signals -

        get into your pajamas
        brush your teeth
        wash your face
        lie down
        relax
        close your eyes
        go to sleep

These pre-sleep rituals will become habit and your body will adapt to getting ready for sleep.

Find out the Root of the Problem.
Many experts feel that determining why we can't sleep may impact our quality of rest. Understanding insomnia will assist us with this. Insomnia is a symptom of another problem, much like a fever or a stomach-ache. Any number of factors can cause it. There are psychological factors, especially during periods of high stress. Problems that are persistent, such as a troubled marriage, a chronically ill child, or an unrewarding career can often contribute to poor sleep. Psychiatric problems may develop. Waking earlier than desired is one of the most common symptoms of depression. If this is a common occurrence with your sleep patterns, seek help.

SLEEP AND ENERGY

Now, how does sleep impact our energy levels? If we haven't received a proper amount of sleep, it affects our daytime schedule. We will feel drowsy, we will have trouble concentrating, and our energy levels will be low. Without the benefits of a good night's sleep our body is fighting to stay awake during the day. We know that the body requires sleep to repair and rebuild. If we don't allow ourselves enough sleep to repair and rebuild, our body will have to do this work during waking hours. **This takes up extra energy leaving our energy reserves depleted.**

If your sleep has been disturbed for more than a month and interferes with the way you feel or function during the day, see your healthcare provider or ask for a referral to a sleep disorder clinic.

THE DO'S AND DON'TS OF A GOOD NIGHT'S SLEEP

The following is a list with some suggestions that may help you get to sleep easier.

DO'S	DON'TS
DO keep a regular schedule. Go to sleep and wake up roughly at the same time every day.	DON'T use alcoholic beverages or street drugs as sedatives.
DO exercise regularly.	DON'T do late evening exercises.
DO have a comfortable bed in a quiet, dark room.	DON'T have your room too cold or too hot.
DO eat a light snack or have a glass of milk if you are hungry before bed.	DON'T eat a heavy meal before retiring and do not snack during the night.
DO keep the bedroom just for sex and sleep; not as an all-purpose activity area.	DON'T try too hard to fall asleep. Get out of bed, do a meditation or something equally relaxing. Return to bed only when you feel sleepy.
DO schedule a relaxation period before going to sleep and establish pre-sleep rituals.	DON'T nap during the day if you are having trouble sleeping during the night. If you are a regular afternoon 'napper', 20 minutes should be your maximum.
DO maintain a regular daytime schedule such as regular morning sun exposure and regular times for eating, taking medications and other activities.	DON'T smoke and/or drink caffeinated beverages within several hours before bed.

OTHER WAYS TO RE-ENERGIZE YOURSELF

Restful "time outs" are a major source of renewed energy.

POWER NAP

More and more studies are proving the benefit of a 15-20 minute Power Nap around 3 p.m. So think about the possibilities of replacing that afternoon coffee break with an afternoon nap break. Even if we don't sleep, the simple fact of taking the time out, totally resting for a full 20 minutes will give us new energy. We will get up refreshed and ready to have our quick power snack and be energized for the rest of the day.

Find a quiet place, if possible turn off the lights (or wear one of those travel sleep masks), turn off the phone, put a "do not disturb" sign on the door and give yourself this gift. They say its best to actually lay down. So, how about that couch in our office or, being realistic, how about bringing a pillow, even a light blanket, and stretching out on the rug. Try it, the benefits will be tremendous.

> **Better set the timer. If this Power Nap goes on too long the benefit is lost as you become sluggish. Oversleeping during the day will disturb your night's sleep, to say nothing of your job.**

MEDITATION

This is the best way we know of to completely relax and refresh our mind. We all need a mental break now and then. We need a way to regain control over our hectic, busy, racing mind. Meditation is a way to do just that. During meditation we not only completely relax our mind, we also get to completely relax our body. Those who meditate regularly tend to be able to more easily manage the stress in their lives, concentrate more easily, and feel more in control of their lives.

Meditation is a passive exercise, which means our job is to do nothing. Our job is to relax every part of our body and to completely let our mind go blank. That, in fact, is the hard part! We can choose a meditation that has a person leading us through the exercise. We simply concentrate on continuous relaxation as we listen to their voice. Or, we can choose quiet music – something specifically made for meditation like Pachelbel's "Canon in D" or Daniel Kobialka's "When You Wish Upon a Star", and simply sit quietly and listen. Some people find that focusing on the flame of a candle works best for them.

> Choose a quiet place either at work or at home where you will not be disturbed. Allow about twenty minutes. Put a clock within easy sight for you to peak at if you wish. Now, relax everything, and just continue to listen. Take a few deep breaths as you get started, then allow yourself to breathe normally. You will find that your mind will interrupt you. This is normal. Simply notice it, and then let it go, and get back to your job of being passive and completely relaxed. If you choose to listen to music or focus on a flame rather than a lead meditation, try repeating a word or phrase over and over quietly in your mind as you exhale. Some people have chosen "peace", "love", "relax", or other words. This will help you to remain focused and not allow your busy mind to interrupt your meditation. When you finish your meditation, take a couple of big breaths, stretch, feel refreshed, re-energized, and ready for the rest of your day.

RELAXATION

This can be anything we choose that causes us to totally lose ourselves. It could be a hobby that we absolutely love to do. It could be a humorous program where we laugh ourselves silly. It could be playing with our children or our grandchildren. It could be reading, art, a hot bubble bath, a massage or yoga.

Whatever we choose, remember our aim is to be relaxed, happy and feeling a sense of satisfaction and pleasure. If what we've chosen starts to cause us stress, causes us to get up tight, we are defeating our purpose. STOP! Change to something that will bring us true relaxation and pleasure. When we love life, we feel energized.

WORRY BUSTING

We seem to be able to find something to worry about throughout our lives. Worry is a huge energy drain. Let's put worry where it belongs "Out of our Lives". A study on people's worries showed

- 40% of the worries people had, never happened
- 30% of the worries were about things in the past
- 12% were about health issues that were needless
- 10% were petty worries
- 8% were actually about something more substantial

4% of the 8% of the more substantial worries were actually **'out of their control'**. If it is 'out of your control', what is the use of worrying about it?
4% of the 8% were worries that were totally or somewhat under their control.

So take this final 4% and apply the **"worry-buster"** technique that we have found to be very effective by following these steps:

1. learn to live life in the present - living one day at a time – (worrying about the past or the future is surely a waste of energy)
2. get all the true facts about a 'worry' – (we may or may not have a clear picture and can be worrying unnecessarily)
3. define this 'worry' clearly in writing – (helps our understanding)
4. determine the worst possible outcome should this 'worry' come true – put it in writing (be very realistic here – don't dramatize – put it into perspective)
5. resolve to accept this worst possible outcome - (let's face 'it', name 'it')
6. begin immediately to improve upon this worst possible outcome – (this important step begins to alleviate our worry as we are already planning how to make it better)

Worries will likely never totally disappear but we can handle them differently. Taking some ACTION, based on clear, factual understanding and acceptance, is a great worry buster and a huge energy gain.

HUMOUR

Yes, we all need to laugh. Find the "bless" in the "mess". Let's learn to laugh at ourselves. What? Is everything serious? It's true, we do tend to take ourselves, our lives, our jobs, and our problems too seriously from time to time.

Laughter is not only fun, it's healthy as it relieves stress and tension, and it is energizing.

Live with JOY in your life.
Find the humour in every day and share it with others.
Invite a friend out to play.
Take a play day.
Have at least one big belly laugh every day.
Watch a comedy show rather than the news before going to bed.
Build more energy into your life through joy and laughter.

COUNT YOUR BLESSINGS

Appreciating what we have rather than continuously wishing for what others have – removes a huge energy drain. Let's learn to count our blessings. In fact, take time right now and write down ten things that you appreciate most in your life.

1.

2.

3.

4.

5.

6.

7.

8.

9.

10.

OXYGEN - DEEP BREATHING

Fresh clean air is a wonderful energizer. Take those fresh air breaks. Get out at noon for that brisk walk. Sometimes it's hard if you work in an area with high vehicle traffic. If possible find a park with lots of greenery.

Take deep breathing breaks throughout the day. Yes, we can 'breathe' anywhere; sitting at our desk, standing in line, driving our car.

> **Breathe in through your nose. First fill your abdomen, then your lower lungs expanding your rib cage, then fill the upper part of your lungs raising your chest and shoulders slightly. This full breath can be done in one smooth continuous inhale. Hold your breath for a few seconds. Then exhale slowly, pulling your abdomen in slightly and relaxing your chest. Take a few regular breaths in between your deep breaths.**

We need to take three or four deep energizing breaths **several times each day**. Deep breathing not only re-energizes our brain and our body, it also releases body tension.

OUR SENSE OF SMELL

Yes we can even energize ourselves through our sense of smell. Let's check out our home, our office. Get rid of the dirt, the old lingering smells. Add fragrances that trigger our energy. Try lemon, peppermint, spearmint, pine, rosemary, eucalyptus, jasmine or basil.

Add a plant or two to help clean the air. After absorbing air contaminants, plants breathe back clean air. Look into purchasing an air purifier.

COLOUR

We can build our energy by adding colour to our living or working space. Reds, yellows, and oranges give off electromagnetic wave bands that actually send impulses of energy to the energy control glands of our brain. Shades of yellow have been proven to have the most energizing effect on people. So think of adding splashes of yellow in areas where we want higher energy.

LIGHT

Turn on the lights, open the curtains and let the sun shine in. We respond to brightness. It energizes us. Get outside into the sunshine every day. The more sunshine we get - the more 'feel-good' chemicals our brain produces.

Indoors, choose warm incandescent light. We could put a lamp with a warm-tinted light bulb on our desk. If we must have fluorescent lights, then we could put in warm-white fluorescent light bulbs, known as daylight bulbs.

NATURAL ENERGY HIGH'S AND LOW'S

By following our many building energy lifestyle choices in this workbook you will be able to maintain a steady energy level. But it is also important to be aware of your own body's natural energy biorhythms. Notice during your day, when you regularly naturally feel more energetic. Whenever possible, capitalize on this natural high by booking your most important meetings, projects, etc, at your highest energy times. Track your energy levels using your **DAILY BUILDING ENERGY RECORD**.

ENERGIZE YOUR WORKSPACE

One of the most important things we have learned is to accept ourselves the way we are. This does not mean that we don't want to continue to learn and grow, but it does mean that we appreciate our own strengths and are not trying to work "differently" to please the style of someone else. That is a big energy drain.

Accept and work with your own best work style. It is important for us to recognize whether we are more 'right brained dominant' or 'left brained dominant'. Those of us who have a 'right' brain dominance may thrive in clutter as our creativity is continuously in high gear. We love to jump from project to project keeping many balls in the air at one time. Conversely, for those of us who have a more 'left' brained dominance we like to have a tidy, finished, and filed workplace with things more orderly and in order. For either of these preferences to try to work in the "other's" environment is a huge energy drain. Many of us want something in between. Whatever your choice/preference – accepting it and working with it, is an energizer of its own.

Personalize your workspace. Surround yourself with things that energize you. Build in some way to relax, to relieve stress, and to maintain energy. Maybe this is a restful picture, a bright colorful picture, a joke, a family picture, a plant, flowers, your goal(s) with supporting sub-goal(s). Whatever it is, have it within easy sight.

Be sure you have taken care of the 'ergonomic' things – taking care of your body, like
- a good chair with adjustable height and adjustable back support (we found the steno chair to work best)
- a foot stool (if you need one) to keep your knees very slightly elevated above your hips
- keep your keyboard low enough that your wrists are not strained in any way
- have your computer screen directly in front of you so that you look straight ahead and slightly lower than eye level – so that there is no strain on your neck or your shoulders
- ensure that there is no reflective glare on your screen
- every five to ten minutes – look beyond your screen for a few seconds to allow your eyes to rest by looking further into the distance
- every hour or so, take shoulder, neck and back stretches to relieve tension
- take those wonderful deep breaths regularly to keep your brain and your body oxygenated

Look around your work environment. Consider all things – colour, lighting, air quality, ergonomics, your own personal work style, your natural energy high's and low's, personalized energizers, and continue to ensure they all support and maintain your energy levels.

STRETCH AT YOUR DESK FOR ENERGY

Many of us in our workplace are sitting at our desk most of our working day. Sometimes we are so busy that we don't take any breaks and even wonder if we took time to get up and go to the bathroom! By the end of the day our muscles are tense; we have sore backs, stiff necks and feel exhausted.

To help keep ourselves energized and release body tension we need to take periodic stretches for energy – and we can do them right at our desks! To help ensure you take timely stretch breaks, set an alarm on your computer, palm organizer or wrist watch for every hour or so. Then push away from your desk and do some deep breathing and simple stretches to release tense muscles and re-energize your body and mind. If your workstation is out in the open and you feel too self-conscious to do these stretches there, do them in the open area of the staff washroom or in the coffee room, just find a place and do them!

Basic tips:
- Breathe naturally during your stretches, don't hold your breath
- Hold each stretch for 15 – 20 seconds or until you feel the tension release
- The stretches for the upper body can be done seated or standing
- If you are standing you can place your feet slightly wider than shoulder width apart for balance, a slight bend in the knees and a 'neutral spine', whatever is comfortable for you
- These are slow "static" or held stretches, try not to bounce during your stretch

Neck, Upper Back and Shoulder Stretches:

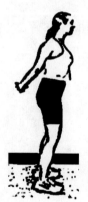

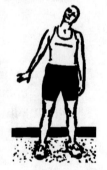

Tilt your head to one side, ear to shoulder, and then with the opposite arm push down and away from your body. This is a great stretch for the muscles in the neck and the top of the shoulder. If you need a further stretch you can put your other hand on your head and pull slightly. Remember to breathe naturally; don't hold your breath while stretching.

Shrug your shoulders up, back and then down and behind to open up the chest. If you can clasp your hands together behind your back that is fine, if not just hold them back to release the tension in the shoulders and chest.

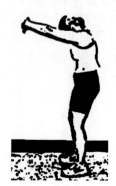

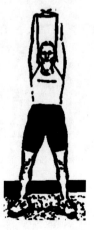

With your hands clasped together reach out in front of your body, tilt your head down, chin to chest and pull your shoulder blades apart. To follow this up you can pull your arms up directly over your head and release the shoulders up as far as you can.

Spine, Lower Back and Hip Stretches:

You can do all of these stretches by sitting up tall at the edge of your chair with both feet flat on the floor with your knees and hips at a 90-degree angle. Use something to help elevate your feet if you need to or adjust your chair.

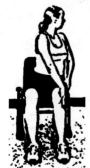

Turn your body to one side with both hands on the outside of your thigh looking behind you. This will allow your spine to laterally rotate and stretch your hard working muscles. Hold, return to center and then repeat on the other side.

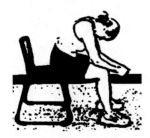

To stretch out the entire spine and release the tension on the discs between the vertebrae, lean forward with your elbows on your knees and drop your head down. Allow your spine to release. If you would like a further stretch you could drop your head and arms all the way down and hang forward. Choose what is most comfortable for you.

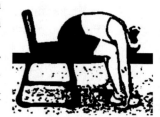

Bring one ankle up and place it on your opposite knee, keeping your body tall. This may be enough of a stretch for you already; you should feel the stretch coming from deep in your hip area. If you need a further stretch, place your palm on your bent knee and slightly push and hold down. Repeat by switching your legs.

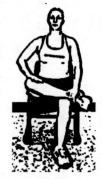

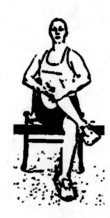

Return to the original position of facing forward with both feet on the ground. Then lift one leg up again, ankle to the opposite knee. This time, lock your hands on the outside of your knee and pull that knee up towards you, still maintaining your 'sitting tall' stance. This will stretch the muscles on the outside of your hip joint. Hold, release and repeat on the other side. If you notice that one side is tighter than the other, it usually indicates which hip you tend to 'sit down into' when you stand.

WATCH WATER WALK WEIGHTS WONDERFUL

WONDERFUL -- is how you will feel!

> Sleep is the repair shop of the body and the brain, the process that most thoroughly restores our vitality after the strains and exertions of life.

My body and my mind are rejuvenated through rest.
I am alert, ENERGIZED, and well rested

My notes on Rejuvenation through Rest are:

Things I am going to do from now on to ensure my body and mind get enough Sleep, Rest, and Relaxation to keep rejuvenated and energized are:

MY NOTES:

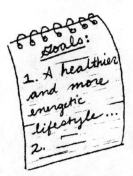

BUILDING

Energy
Nutrition
Exercise
Rest and Relaxation
GOALS
YOU

SECTION FIVE

COMMIT TO A GOAL

THAT IS RIGHT FOR YOU

To turn a wish into a REALITY, we need to:
write it down,
make it realistic and do-able for ourselves,
put a time frame on it,
tell others and solicit their support,
do it, and
celebrate our successes.

LEARNING OBJECTIVE

After reading this Section and completing all the exercises, you will

- **begin to develop a personal action plan for your own journey to a healthier and more ENERGETIC lifestyle**

ATTITUDE

Our attitude and our commitment to loving and caring for ourselves is critically important as we decide how to build some BETTER CHOICES into our lives.

"I am worth it. I can do it." Repeat these statements to yourself often and meaningfully. Have a plan of action, write your goal, make your commitment, and get started. You can always make adjustments as you go along.

You have nothing to lose and everything to gain. Build your ENERGY by choosing quality food, drinking sufficient water, building physical activity into your day, and getting sufficient rest.

We've shared as much as we could in this book – now IT'S UP TO YOU. Read this story about ATTITUDE and make your choices.

A STORY ABOUT *ATTITUDE*

Michael is the kind of guy you love to love. He is always in a good mood and always has something positive to say. When someone would ask him how he was doing, he would reply, "If I were any better, I'd have to be twins".

He was a natural motivator. If an employee was having a bad day, Michael was there, telling the employee how to look on the positive side of the situation. Seeing this style really made me curious. So, one day I went up to Michael and asked him, "I don't get it! You can't be a positive person all of the time. How do you do it?"

Michael replied, "Each morning I wake up and say to myself, you have two choices today. You can choose to be in a good mood or you can choose to be in a bad mood. *I choose to be in a good mood*. Each time something bad happens, I can choose to be a victim or I can choose to learn from it. *I choose to learn from it.* Every time someone comes to me complaining, I can choose to accept their complaining or I can point out the positive side of life. *I choose the positive side of life."*

"Yeah, right, it's not that easy," I protested.

"Yes, it is", Michael said. "Life is all about choices. When you cut away all the junk, every situation is a choice.

> **YOU choose how you react to situations.**
> **YOU choose how people affect your mood.**
> **YOU choose to be in a good mood or a bad mood.**
> **The bottom line is: It's your choice how you live your life."**

I reflected on what Michael said. Soon thereafter, I left my job to start my own business. Michael and I lost touch, but I often thought about him when I made a choice about life instead of reacting to it.

Several years later, I heard that Michael was involved in a serious accident, falling some 60 feet from a communications tower. After 18 hours of surgery and weeks of intensive care, Michael was released from hospital with rods placed in his back. I saw Michael about six months after the accident. When I asked him how he was, he replied. "If I were any better, I'd be twins. Wanna see my scars?"

I declined to see his wounds, but I did ask him what had gone through his mind as the accident took place. "The first thing that went through my mind was the well being of my soon to be born daughter," Michael replied. "Then, as I lay on the ground, I remembered that I had two choices: I could choose to live or I could choose to die. *I chose to live."*

"Weren't you scared? Did you lose consciousness?" I asked.

Michael continued, "...the paramedics were great. They kept telling me I was going to be fine. But when they wheeled me into the ER and I saw the expressions on the faces of the doctors and nurses, I got really scared. In their eyes, I read 'he's a dead man'. I knew I needed to take action."

"What did you do?" I asked.

"Well, there was a big burly nurse shouting questions at me," said Michael. "She asked if I was allergic to anything. 'Yes!' I replied. The doctors and nurses stopped working as they waited for my reply. I took a deep breath and yelled, 'GRAVITY'. Over their laughter, I told them, *I am choosing to live*. Operate on me as if I am alive, not dead."

Michael lived, thanks to the skill of his doctors and because of his amazing attitude. I learned from him that every day we have the choice to live life fully.

Anonymous

ATTITUDE is everything.
So, the most important thing you can do to improve your health
and bring more energy into your life is to
choose to do it.

TEN TIPS TO BUILDING ENERGY
IT'S ALL ABOUT CHOICES

1. **Eat Early - Eat Often** - Keep your body and your brain energized with small meals and snacks throughout the day.

2. **Eat for Energy** - Stay full and energized over longer periods of time. Eat complex carbohydrates and protein at every meal and snack. Keep your portions small and balanced at ¾ carbohydrates to ¼ protein.

3. **Eat Light** - Trim some fat from your diet. Choose low or no fat products.

4. **Energize With Water** - Make WATER your drink of choice. Don't feed your thirst. Ensure you keep your body well hydrated throughout the day.

5. **Keep Moving** - Build daily energy by building in several segments of physical activity throughout your day. Get creative.

6. **Breathe Deeply** - Keep your body and your brain oxygenated and stay energized.

7. **Stay Flexible - Stay Strong** - Be able to reach, bend, lift, carry, walk, and play all your life.

8. **Rest, Relax, Rejuvenate** - Give your body the Rest that it needs. Set yourself up for the deep, complete, restful sleep that your body needs to repair and rejuvenate.

9. **Choose Your ATTITUDE** - Take pleasure in life, use humour and find joy in the things that you do.

10. **Make a Commitment to Yourself** - Set your goals. Make them do-able and personally meaningful.

ABOVE ALL ELSE, LOVE AND CARE FOR YOURSELF

THE ENERGY EQUATION REVISITED

Your **Energy Equation** is up to you.
We've discovered ways that help us increase our energy.
We've also looked at how we can be draining our own energy.

Now look seriously at how you can build **your own ENERGY EQUATION** and build more energy into your life.

Reflect back on everything you have read and learned from this Workbook,
and now choose things that are "right" for you and build on your -

ENERGY EQUATION.

+ PLUS + ENERGY GAINS	- MINUS - ENERGY DRAINS

= EQUALS =

"SURPLUS ENERGY FOR YOU"

ENERGY MIND MAP

My ENERGY MIND MAP PLAN for change is: (*Check back to all your Five W's Pages*)

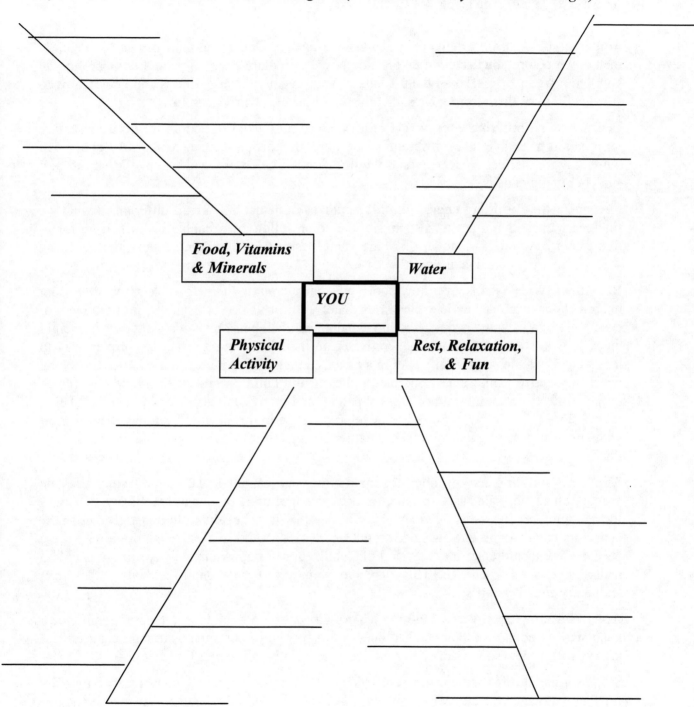

GUIDELINES TO SUSTAINED ENERGY

Making any change in our lives is a process; we want you to understand that each day is a new day. The following are some guidelines to consider when you are implementing changes to your life to increase your energy levels.

1. **Make personal commitments to the energy equation.** Don't wait until you have an energy melt down before you decide to take action to create a more energetic you. Look carefully at your energy equation, take an honest look at your negative energy drains and decide how to slowly eliminate them from your equation and go for the positive surplus.

2. **Learn proven building energy techniques.** Once mobilized to action, we need to acquire information to enable us to differentiate between the techniques that will work for us, and those that are ineffective. Understand the tips of building energy and play with them to best suit your energy needs.

3. **Recognize that building energy is unique for each of us.** We are all different in what we find energizing. If it's fun upbeat music, the color yellow or a bubble bath, then go for it. Remember our body is unique, there are some basics to the building energy tips, but find what works for you and take action.

4. **Be patient.** When we discover how poorly we manage our own energy levels, we often want to correct our perceived deficiencies immediately. Unfortunately, this is seldom possible. For example, all of us know people who have undertaken fad diets and lost a great deal of weight quickly. However, these people generally regain their lost weight. The only proven way to lose weight is to do so gradually, eating a balanced diet with reduced caloric intake and being physically active. This same principle applies to the building energy tips. The benefits of changed lifestyles are not immediately apparent, and improvements in health and well-being accrue slowly. Therefore, we need to develop patience in our efforts. You may want to start with one change, going to bed one hour earlier for example, and then try an additional energy builder.

5. **Approach building energy one step at a time.** We cannot make major lasting lifestyle changes on a wholesale basis. Instead, we need to concentrate on one or two lifestyle changes for a minimum trial basis of **forty days**. After this time, evaluate the change these new behaviors have had on our lives and to our energy levels. If we elect to continue with these changes, we should enter into a period of stabilization for approximately two months before undertaking another change. This way we gain new permanent life habits rather than temporary added changes.

6. **Accept building energy as a life-long learning process.** A book or a seminar may provide a good starting point, but the overall process must be one of continual learning because there always will be new sources of energy builders, especially in the nutrition area.

7. **Stop waging battles we cannot win.** Many of us cause ourselves unnecessary stress by fighting every stressor that comes our way. We must learn to distinguish between the battles that are worth waging and those that are not. Spending time on negative issues is a great waste of our energy; turn your energy into a positive and stop fighting the fights not worth the negative energy.

8. **Confront change and energy with a positive attitude.** From the attitude story you have just read you can see how remaining positive will create amazing energy. Take a lesson from Michael and stay positive. Taking initiatives, reaching out and confronting our environments in a positive way, are necessary to effect specific lifestyle changes.

9. **Take calculated risks.** Other people often do not want or expect us to change because they are used to our behaving in certain ways. You may be seen as a bit strange when you are taking an energy break rather than a coffee break, doing exercises at your work station, opting to take the stairs instead of the elevator etc. Keep true to yourself and your commitments, who knows others may take notice of your new found fountain of energy!

10. **Effect the easier lifestyle changes before we attempt the more difficult ones.** For example, some of us may want to try to start drinking more water before we join a gym to exercise 3 – 5 times a week. Early success experiences help to build momentum and to lessen the difficulty of effecting later changes.

11. **Expect to succeed.** Expectations become self-fulfilling; if we expect to succeed, our chances of doing so are much higher than if we expect to fail. An optimistic approach is not difficult to maintain if we follow the preceding guidelines of effecting changes one step at a time, taking risks, and building on successes.

12. **Remain open to new information.** Once we have adopted lifestyle changes and have become accustomed to them, it is natural to start taking them for granted and stop noticing and actively acquiring further information about them. When this process occurs, we cease to learn and tend to lose our objectivity about our new habits. It is a good idea to remain open and flexible about lifestyle changes so that further transitions, should they be appropriate, can be made easily.

13. **Build and use our support networks.** Lifestyle changes, both on and off the job, are difficult to make and maintain. Often we can facilitate these changes by soliciting the help or guidance of others. Let those around you know that you are making a conscious choice to become more energetic. Their support will be greatly appreciated in your goal setting objectives.

> *In summary, remember that change is a process, take one day at a time, surround yourself with happy positive people and find the things you love to do and do them!*

BECOMING A HEALTHIER – MORE ENERGETIC YOU

Think over everything we have reviewed in this book. Building more energy into your life means making some lifestyle changes. You have completed your Energy Mind Map, your Energy Equation and you have read over our Guidelines to Sustained Energy. Now it is time to make the commitment and do it.

Use YOUR DAILY BUILDING ENERGY RECORD to help keep you on track.

You have the power!

Within the next six months, I will put more energy into my life by:

> **"Life is a banquet and most fools are starving to death."**
> Anonymous

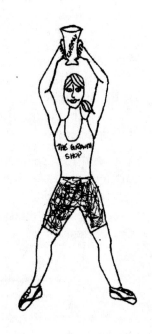

CONGRATULATIONS!

Even if you are on the right track, if you never move, you'll still get run over by the train.

YOUR DAILY BUILDING ENERGY RECORD

As you begin to take control of your FOOD CHOICES, you need to help yourself until this new behaviour becomes a habit. So for at least one month, and whenever you need to again, track everything you eat, note your comments, forgive any slips and just keep moving toward a HEALTHIER, MORE ENERGETIC YOU.

Time	Food (include serving size) Track CARBOHYDRATES (C), FATS (F) & PROTEIN (P) in the next box	C F P	Degree of Hunger 0-4	Water Intake	Situation FOOD - place/activity EXERCISE – Describe	ENERGY LEVEL 0-4 COMMENTS

PLEASE copy and use YOUR DAILY BUILDING ENERGY RECORD until you've changed your habits. Repeat if necessary.

YOUR DAILY BUILDING ENERGY RECORD

As you begin to take control of your FOOD CHOICES, you need to help yourself until this new behaviour becomes a habit. So for at least one month, and whenever you need to again, track everything you eat, note your comments, forgive any slips and just keep moving toward a HEALTHIER, MORE ENERGETIC YOU.

Time	Food (include serving size) Track CARBOHYDRATES (C), FATS (F) & PROTEIN (P) in the next box	C F P	Degree of Hunger 0-4	Water Intake	Situation FOOD - place/activity EXERCISE – Describe	ENERGY LEVEL 0-4 COMMENTS

PLEASE XEROX and use YOUR DAILY BUILDING ENERGY RECORD until you've changed your habits. Repeat if necessary.

BIBLIOGRAPHY OF RESOURCES

Berkeley Wellness Letter, The University of California, the newsletter of nutrition, fitness, and stress management, published in association with the School of Public Health, P.O. Box 420148, Palm Coast, Florida 32142

Exercise Intensity and Body Fat Loss, National Strength and Conditioning Journal, V. 14, #6, 1992, Susan N. Puhl, and Kristine Clark

Fat Burning: Getting Down to the Basics, Article from FITNESS Management Magazine, March 1996, Barbara A. Brehm, Ed. D.

Fitness Theory Manual, Alberta Fitness Leadership Association, 2000

Guidelines for Exercise Testing and Prescription, American College of Sports Medicine 1991, Philadelphia, P. A., Lea and Febiger

Insomnia -The Inability to Fall Asleep or Stay Asleep, A Wellness booklet from the Canadian Sleep Society- 1997

Low Fat Living, Rodale Press, Inc., Emmaus, Pennsylvania, 1996 - Robert K. Cooper, Ph.D., with Leslie L. Cooper,

Nutrition Action Health Letter, Nutrition Action Health Letter, Centre for Science in the Public Interest (CSPI), P.O. Box 70373, Toronto Station A, Toronto, Ontario, M5W 2X5, founded 1971, an independent, non-profit consumer health group. www.cspinet.org

Picture Perfect Weight Loss, Rodale Press, Inc, Emmaus, Pennsylvania, 2000 - Howard M. Shapiro, M.D.

Resistance Training- A Manual for Fitness Leaders, Ministry of Tourism and Recreation Printed by the Queen's Printer for Ontario, Toronto, Canada, 1992 Government of Ontario

Sleep Wake Disorders Canada (SWDC), 5055, 3080 Young Street, Toronto, Ontario, M4N 3N1(416) 483-9654 or 1-800-387-9253 e-mail swdc@globalserve.net

Sleep Well Tonight – *Sure-fire solutions to a good night's rest*, Sterling Publishing Co., Inc., 387 Park Avenue South, New York, N.Y. 10016-8810, 1998 by Harriet Griffey

The Canadian Sleep Society (CSS), 5055, 3080 Young Street, Toronto, Ontario, M4N 3N1 (416) 483-6260

The Energy Edge, Life Line Press, an Eagle Publishing Company, One Massachusetts Avenue NW, Washington, DC, 2001, 1999 - Pamela Smith, R.D.

The Gylcemic Index Diet, Random House Canada, Richard Gallop, www.randomhouse.ca

The New Fit or Fat, Houghton Mufflin Company, 2 Park Street, Boston, Massachusetts 92108, 1991 by Covert Bailey

What to do When you Can't Sleep, A brochure developed as a public service by Wake Up Canada! - Sleep/Wake Disorders Canada

YMCA Weight Training Instructor's Manual- Copyright 1986- The Regional Council of Young Men's Christian Associations of Canada, Toronto

You Count, Calories Don't, Hyperion Press, 300 Wales Avenue, Winnipeg, MB., R2M 2S9, 1992 - Linda Omichinski, B.Sc., (F.Sc.), R.D.

You Don't Have to go Home from Work Exhausted, Bowen and Rogers, P.O. Box 64784, Dallas, Texas, 75206, 1990 by Ann McGee-Cooper with Duane Trammell and Barbara Lau

Your Body's Many Cries for Water, Global Health Solutions, Inc., P.O. Box 3189, Falls Church, VA 22043, (703) 848-2333, Fax 703-848-2334, 1997 –F. Batmanghelidj, M.D.

ABOUT THE MOTHER AND DAUGHTER TEAM OF AUTHORS

Beverly M. Richardson

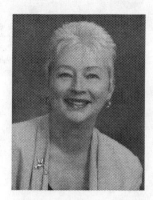

Bev Richardson is the owner and operator of **Richardson Enterprises** and is the Design Consultant with **The Growth Shop.** Bev has been working in adult education for over twenty years. Most of those years were spent with the Organization and Staff Development Agency, Manitoba Provincial Government. During that time, she researched, designed, delivered and evaluated many training programs. She also found herself filling roles as coordinator, supervisor, manager and consultant. Since 1998, Bev has been delivering and designing courses through her own business and as a partner with **The Growth Shop.**

Bev holds two three-year Certificates from the University of Manitoba, one in Human Resource Management and one in Adult and Continuing Education and is a qualified Myers-Briggs trainer through Psychometrics Canada, Alberta.

Bev resides in Winnipeg, Manitoba with her husband Jim. She is now semi-retired spending more time seeking leisurely pursuits such as summers at her cottage on Lake Winnipeg, golfing, traveling to all parts of the world and spending time with her five granddaughters.

Wendy A. Bodnar

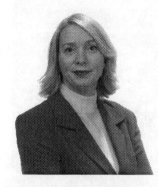

Wendy Bodnar is the owner and operator of **The Growth Shop** a company that designs and delivers sessions in personal and professional growth. She is a dynamic presenter and her humorous style gets results! She has facilitated stress and energy workshops and talks across Canada to hundreds of participants in all levels of government, hospitals, small and large businesses. She was featured in the *Edmonton Journal* and the *Edmontonian* newspapers and was a regular guest on CBC's 'Bodytalk'.

Wendy specializes in the delivery of **Managing Workplace and Personal Stress, Stress Busters, Stress Bites** and, **Building Energy** workshops and in keynote presentations. Her keynotes include: **'Stress and the Caveman'**, **'Stress is a Six Letter Word: Six Proven Strategies to Master Stress'**, **Building Energy in a Low Energy World'**, **'Healthy Mind, Healthy Body, Healthy Bottom Line'** and the **'Love Story of the Hogar'**. Wendy has a Bachelor of Physical Education degree, has coordinated provincial fitness leadership programs and is a member of the Canadian Association of Professional Speakers. Contact Wendy at www.thegrowthshop.com.

Wendy resides in Edmonton, Alberta, with her husband Paul and has three daughters Monica, Anastasia and Sarah.